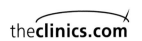

VETERINARY CLINICS

OF NORTH AMERICA

Small Animal Practice

Emerging and Reemerging Viruses
of Dogs and Cats

GUEST EDITORS
Sanjay Kapil, DVM, MS, PhD
Catherine G. Lamm, DVM

July 2008 • Volume 38 • Number 4

SAUNDERS

An Imprint of Elsevier, Inc.
PHILADELPHIA   LONDON   TORONTO   MONTREAL   SYDNEY   TOKYO

W.B. SAUNDERS COMPANY
A Division of Elsevier Inc.

Elsevier, Inc., 1600 John F. Kennedy Blvd., Suite 1800, Philadelphia, PA 19103-2899

http://www.vetsmall.theclinics.com

VETERINARY CLINICS OF NORTH AMERICA:	**Volume 38, Number 4**
SMALL ANIMAL PRACTICE	**ISSN 0195-5616**
July 2008	**ISBN-13: 978-1-4160-6373-5**
Editor: John Vassallo; j.vassallo@elsevier.com	**ISBN-10: 1-4160-6373-0**

The ideas and opinions expressed in *Veterinary Clinics of North America: Small Animal Practice* do not necessarily reflect those of the Publisher. The Publisher does not assume any responsibility for any injury and/or damage to persons or property arising out of or related to any use of the material contained in this periodical. The reader is advised to check the appropriate medical literature and the product information currently provided by the manufacturer of each drug to be administered to verify the dosage, the method and duration of administration, or contraindications. It is the responsibility of the treating physician or other health care professional, relying on independent experience and knowledge of the patient, to determine drug dosages and the best treatment for the patient. Mention of any product in this issue should not be construed as endorsement by the contributors, editors, or the Publisher of the product or manufacturers' claims.

Veterinary Clinics of North America: Small Animal Practice (ISSN 0195-5616) is published bimonthly (For Post Office use only: volume 38 issue 4 of 6) by Elsevier Inc., 360 Park Avenue South, New York, NY 10010-1710. Months of issue are January, March, May, July, September, and November. Business and Editorial offices: 1600 John F. Kennedy Blvd., Suite 1800, Philadelphia, PA 19103-2899. Customer Service Office: 6277 Sea Harbor Drive, Orlando, FL 32887-4800. Periodicals postage paid at New York, NY and additional mailing offices. Subscription prices are $206.00 per year for US individuals, $327.00 per year for US institutions, $103.00 per year for US students and residents, $273.00 per year for Canadian individuals, $410.00 per year for Canadian institutions, $285.00 per year for international individuals, $410.00 per year for international institutions and $140.00 per year for Canadian and foreign students/residents. To receive student/resident rate, orders must be accompanied by name of affiliated institution, date of term, and the *signature* of program/residency coordinator on institution letterhead. Orders will be billed at individual rate until proof of status is received. Foreign air speed delivery is included in all *Clinics* subscription prices. All prices are subject to change without notice. **POSTMASTER**: Send address changes to *Veterinary Clinics of North America: Small Animal Practice*, Elsevier Periodicals Customer Service, 6277 Sea Harbor Drive, Orlando, FL 32887-4800. Customer Service: 1-800-654-2452 (US). From outside the United States, call 1-407-563-6020. Fax: 1-407-363-9661. E-mail: JournalsCustomerService-usa@elsevier.com.

Veterinary Clinics of North America: Small Animal Practice is also published in Japanese by Inter Zoo Publishing Co., Ltd., Aoyama Crystal-Bldg 5F, 3-5-12 Kitaaoyama, Minato-ku, Tokyo 107-0061, Japan.

Reprints: For copies of 100 or more, of articles in this publication, please contact the Commercial Reprints Department, Elsevier Inc., 360 Park Avenue South, New York, New York 10010-1710. Tel. (212) 633-3813 Fax: (212) 462-1935, email: reprints@elsevier.com.

Veterinary Clinics of North America: Small Animal Practice is covered in *Current Contents/Agriculture, Biology and Environmental Sciences, Science Citation Index, ASCA, MEDLINE/PubMed (Index Medicus), Excerpta Medica,* and *BIOSIS*.

Printed in the United States of America.

ELSEVIER
SAUNDERS

VETERINARY CLINICS
SMALL ANIMAL PRACTICE

Emerging and Reemerging Viruses of Dogs and Cats

GUEST EDITORS

SANJAY KAPIL, DVM, MS, PhD, Diplomate, American College of Veterinary Microbiologists (Virology and Immunology); Diplomate, American College of Veterinary Medicine; Professor of Clinical Virology, Oklahoma Animal Disease Diagnostic Laboratory, Oklahoma State University, Center for Veterinary Health Sciences, Stillwater, Oklahoma

CATHERINE G. LAMM, DVM, Diplomate, American College of Veterinary Pathologists; Assistant Professor of Veterinary Anatomic Pathology, Oklahoma Animal Disease Diagnostic Laboratory, Oklahoma State University, Center for Veterinary Health Sciences, Stillwater, Oklahoma

CONTRIBUTORS

JOE BROWNLIE, BVSc, PhD, DSc, FRCPath, FRCVS, Diplomate, European College of Veterinary Pathologists; Professor of Veterinary Pathology, Department of Pathology and Infectious Diseases, The Royal Veterinary College, Hatfield, United Kingdom

CANIO BUONAVOGLIA, DVM, Full Professor, Department of Animal Health and Wellbeing, Faculty of Veterinary Medicine, University of Bari, Valenzano, Bari, Italy

KYEONG-OK CHANG, DVM, PhD, Diagnostic Medicine and Pathobiology, College of Veterinary Medicine, Kansas State University, Manhattan, Kansas

NICOLA DECARO, DVM, Associate Professor, Department of Animal Health and Wellbeing, Faculty of Veterinary Medicine, University of Bari, Valenzano, Bari, Italy

EDWARD J. DUBOVI, PhD, Professor, Department of Population Medicine and Diagnostic Sciences, Animal Health Diagnostic Center, College of Veterinary Medicine, Cornell University, Ithaca, New York

STEPHEN P. DUNHAM, BVSc, PhD, CertSAC, MRCVS, Lecturer in Veterinary Virology, Division of Veterinary Infection and Immunity, Institute of Comparative Medicine, University of Glasgow, Faculty of Veterinary Medicine, Glasgow, United Kingdom

GABRIELLA ELIA, DVM, Associate Professor, Department of Animal Health and Wellbeing, Faculty of Veterinary Medicine, University of Bari, Bari, Italy

KERSTIN ERLES, DrMedVet, Lecturer in Veterinary Microbiology, Department of Pathology and Infectious Diseases, The Royal Veterinary College, Hatfield, United Kingdom

JAMES F. EVERMANN, PhD, Professor of Infectious Diseases, Department of Veterinary Clinical Sciences, Washington Animal Disease Diagnostic Laboratory, College of Veterinary Medicine, Washington State University, Pullman, Washington

ZHEN F. FU, DVM, PhD, Professor, Department of Pathology, College of Veterinary Medicine, University of Georgia, Athens, Georgia

ELIZABETH GRAHAM, MVB, MVM, PhD, MRCVS, Registrar in Infectious Diseases, Companion Animal Diagnostics, Division of Pathological Sciences, Institute of Comparative Medicine, University of Glasgow, Faculty of Veterinary Medicine, Glasgow, United Kingdom

BILL JOHNSON, DVM, Diplomate, American College of Veterinary Pathologists; Professor of Pathology, Oklahoma Animal Disease Diagnostic Laboratory, Oklahoma State University, Center for Veterinary Health Sciences, Stillwater, Oklahoma

SANJAY KAPIL, DVM, MS, PhD, Diplomate, American College of Veterinary Microbiologists (Virology and Immunology); Diplomate, American College of Veterinary Medicine; Professor of Clinical Virology, Oklahoma Animal Disease Diagnostic Laboratory, Oklahoma State University, Center for Veterinary Health Sciences, Stillwater, Oklahoma

MELISSA KENNEDY, DVM, PhD, Diplomate, American College of Veterinary Medicine; Associate Professor of Virology, Department of Comparative Medicine, College of Veterinary Medicine, Veterinary Teaching Hospital, University of Tennessee, Knoxville, Tennessee

YI KUANG, MD, Graduate Student, Department of Pathology, College of Veterinary Medicine, University of Georgia, Athens, Georgia

SARAH N. LACKAY, MS, Graduate Student, Department of Pathology, College of Veterinary Medicine, University of Georgia, Athens, Georgia

CATHERINE G. LAMM, DVM, Diplomate, American College of Veterinary Pathologists; Assistant Professor of Veterinary Anatomic Pathology, Oklahoma Animal Disease Diagnostic Laboratory, Oklahoma State University, Center for Veterinary Health Sciences, Stillwater, Oklahoma

VITO MARTELLA, DVM, Associate Professor, Department of Animal Health and Wellbeing, Faculty of Veterinary Medicine, University of Bari, Valenzano, Bari, Italy

DAVID SCOTT MCVEY, DVM, PhD, Diplomate, American College of Veterinary Medicine; Professor of Clinical Microbiology, Nebraska Veterinary Diagnostic Center, Department of Veterinary and Biomedical Sciences, College of Agriculture and Natural Resources, University of Nebraska-Lincoln, Lincoln, Nebraska

BRADLEY L. NJAA, DVM, MVSc, Diplomate, American College of Veterinary Pathologists; Associate Professor of Veterinary Pathology, Department of Veterinary Pathobiology, Center for Veterinary Health Sciences, Oklahoma State University, Stillwater, Oklahoma

JOHN S.L. PARKER, BVMS, PhD, Department of Microbiology and Immunology, Baker Institute for Animal Health, College of Veterinary Medicine, Cornell University, Ithaca, New York

PATRICIA A. PESAVENTO, DVM, PhD, Diplomate, American College of Veterinary Pathologists; Department of Pathology, Microbiology, and Immunology, School of Veterinary Medicine, University of California, Davis, Davis, California

GRANT B. REZABEK, MPH, DVM, Assistant Professor, Oklahoma Animal Disease Diagnostic Laboratory, Oklahoma State University, Center for Veterinary Health Sciences, Stillwater, Oklahoma

TERESA YEARY, PhD, Center for Veterinary Biologics, Veterinary Services, Animal and Plant Health Inspection Service, United States Department of Agriculture, Ames, Iowa

ELSEVIER
SAUNDERS

VETERINARY CLINICS
SMALL ANIMAL PRACTICE

Emerging and Reemerging Viruses of Dogs and Cats

CONTENTS   VOLUME 38 • NUMBER 4 • JULY 2008

In this article, the authors are specifically concerned with the timely and accurate detection of emerging diseases of small animals that are viral in origin. Veterinarians are bound to encounter emerging viruses in their practice. The problem is unavoidable, because viruses are highly mutagenic. Even the immune response dictates the nature of virus that evolves in a host. If the clinical signs and diagnostic methods fail to correlate, the veterinarian should work with the diagnostic laboratory to solve the diagnostic puzzle.

Caliciviridae are small, nonenveloped, positive-stranded RNA viruses. Much of our understanding of the molecular biology of the caliciviruses has come from the study of the naturally occurring animal caliciviruses. In particular, many studies have focused on the molecular virology of feline calicivirus (FCV), which reflects its importance as a natural pathogen of cats. FCVs demonstrate a remarkable capacity for high genetic, antigenic, and clinical diversity; "outbreak" vaccine resistant strains occur frequently. This article updates the reader on the current status of clinical behavior and pathogenesis of FCV.

Vaccine-based prophylaxis has greatly helped to keep distemper disease under control. Notwithstanding, the incidence of canine distemper virus (CDV)–related disease in canine populations throughout the world seems to have increased in the past decades, and several episodes of CDV disease in vaccinated animals have been reported, with nationwide proportions in some cases. Increasing surveillance should be pivotal to identify new CDV variants and to understand the dynamics of CDV epidemiology. In addition, it is important to evaluate whether the efficacy of the vaccine against these new strains may somehow be affected.

Canine adenoviruses (CAVs) and canine herpesvirus (CHV) are pathogens of dogs that have been known for several decades. The two distinct types of CAVs, type 1 and type 2, are responsible for infectious canine hepatitis and infectious tracheobronchitis, respectively. In the present article, the currently available literature on CAVs and CHV is reviewed, providing a meaningful update on the epidemiologic, pathogenetic, clinical, diagnostic, and prophylactic aspects of the infections caused by these important pathogens.

Infectious respiratory disease in dogs is a constant challenge because of the involvement of several pathogens and environmental factors. Canine respiratory coronavirus (CRCoV) is a new coronavirus of dogs, which is widespread in North America, Japan, and several European countries. CRCoV has been associated with respiratory disease, particularly in kenneled dog populations. The virus is genetically and antigenically distinct from enteric canine coronavirus; therefore, specific tests are required for diagnosis.

In 2004, the isolation of an influenza virus from racing greyhounds changed the point of reference for discussions about influenza virus in dogs. A virus isolated from greyhounds did not have its origin in a previously described human influenza virus but came from a virus with an equine history. More significantly, evidence emerged to indicate that the virus was capable of transmission from dog to dog. This virus is now referred to as canine influenza virus (CIV) and is the focus of this review. Because the history of CIV is relatively short, the impact of this virus on canine health is yet to be determined.

Parvovirus infects a wide variety of species. The rapid evolution, environmental resistance, high dose of viral shedding, and interspecies transmission have made some strains of parvovirus infection difficult to control within domestic animal populations. Some parvoviruses in companion animals, such as canine parvovirus (CPV) 1 and feline

animals, however. This latter possibility represents the greater risk. Because this represents an ongoing threat, research and development should continue to maximize broad efficacy and effectiveness in addition to safety. To achieve these goals, the research and development effort should evaluate newer available technologies that may also reduce any barriers to use and availability.

The use of biologics in veterinary medicine has been of tremendous value in safeguarding our animal populations from debilitating and oftentimes fatal disease. This article reviews the principles of vaccination and the extensive quality control efforts that are incorporated into preparing the vaccines. Examples of adverse events that have occurred in the past and how enhanced vigilance at the level of the veterinarian and the veterinary diagnostic laboratory help to curtail these events are discussed. Emphasis on understanding the ecology of viral infections in dogs and cats is introduced, together with the concepts of the potential role of vaccines in interspecies spread of viruses.

VETERINARY CLINICS
SMALL ANIMAL PRACTICE

ELSEVIER
SAUNDERS

FORTHCOMING ISSUES

RECENT ISSUES

Vet Clin Small Anim 38 (2008) xiii–xiv

VETERINARY CLINICS
SMALL ANIMAL PRACTICE

Preface

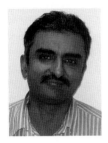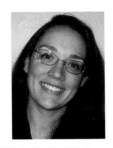

Sanjay Kapil, DVM, MS, PhD
Catherine G. Lamm, DVM
Guest Editors

To our fellow veterinarians, virologists, diagnosticians, and veterinary students: it is our pleasure to bring to you the latest practical developments in companion animal viruses. Viruses are obligate pathogens, and they are evolving constantly to adapt to their hosts. Viruses are challenged by changes in host immunity, vaccination, and host genetics. Mutants arise during infection cycles in an effort to adapt to challenges, and the viral genome is prone to errors. A clinical specimen contains quasi-species of viruses that are selected by the host immune and tissue environments. The mutation rates of RNA and single-stranded DNA viruses can be extremely high, which can lead to vaccine failures.

In this issue of the *Veterinary Clinics of North America: Small Animal Practice*, we have requested the authors assemble the latest developments in the understanding of companion animal viruses. Several of these authors have contributed to the original discovery and description of new viral diseases that affect various organ systems in companion animals. This issue is organized so that small animal veterinarians can easily find the latest information about clinical signs, diagnosis, epidemiology, vaccination, unique features of novel viruses, and management of viral diseases. Throughout the articles, the authors have shared their wisdom on matters of practical concern and relevance to veterinarians. Because the topics are current, this edition will be a useful supplement to a good textbook in small animal viral diseases.

We thank the editors of Elsevier/Saunders, especially John Vassallo, for their help in bringing this issue to you. Dr. Sanjay Kapil thanks his mentor, Professor S. M. Goyal at the University of Minnesota in St. Paul, Minnesota, and Cathy Lamm thanks Dr. Bradley Njaa at Cornell University in New York

0195-5616/08/$ – see front matter
doi:10.1016/j.cvsm.2008.03.007

and Linda Munson at the University of California, Davis for their constant encouragement and guidance. Best wishes!

Sanjay Kapil, DVM, MS, PhD
Catherine G. Lamm, DVM
Oklahoma Animal Disease Diagnostic Laboratory
Oklahoma State University for
Veterinary Health Sciences
Farm and Ridge Road
Stillwater, OK 74074, USA

E-mail addresses: sanjay.kapil@okstate.edu;
cathy.lamm@okstate.edu

Vet Clin Small Anim 38 (2008) 755–774

VETERINARY CLINICS
SMALL ANIMAL PRACTICE

Diagnostic Investigation of Emerging Viruses of Companion Animals

Sanjay Kapil, DVM, MS, PhD[a],*, Teresa Yeary, PhD[b], Bill Johnson, DVM[a]

[a]Oklahoma Animal Disease Diagnostic Laboratory, Oklahoma State University, Center for Veterinary Health Sciences, Farm and Ridge Road, Stillwater, OK 74074, USA
[b]Center for Veterinary Biologics, Veterinary Services, Animal and Plant Health Inspection Service, United States Department of Agriculture, 1800 Dayton Avenue, Ames, IA 50010, USA

C linicians and laboratorians are usually the first to detect most outbreaks of emerging diseases in animals. Much attention is rightfully given to emerging diseases of commercial food animals; however, small animal practitioners also have an obligation to be vigilant to the possibility that new and devastating viral diseases might emerge that infect the companion animals in their charge. Canine parvovirus (CPV) type 2, emerged in 1978 and spread worldwide within less than 2 years [1]. In 2001, a new antigenic type, CPV-2c, was reported in Italy [2], which has since caused outbreaks in Western Europe, Asia, South America, and the United States [3] because current vaccines offer no protection for this type. In this article, the authors are specifically concerned with the timely and accurate detection of emerging diseases of small animals that are viral in origin. The term *emerging virus* is defined broadly and includes these categories:

- Variants of a known virus that has gained enhanced virulence or that is able to infect completely vaccinated animals
- A known virus that has reappeared in the population after a decline in incidence
- Novel or previously unidentified viral agents detected for the first time because of improved diagnostic capabilities
- "Mystery diseases" with large numbers of naive animals involved that are caused by previously uncharacterized viruses

Spread of an emerging virus among small companion animals is multifactorial and includes animal health and sanitation practices; migration of a pathogen from a wild reservoir to domestic animals because of changes in populations, trade, climate, land use, and the introduction of invasive species (eg, plant, animal, insect); and, finally, globalization, as was the case with West Nile virus (WNV). Emerging viral infections may take a heavy toll on the health of cats

*Corresponding author. E-mail address: sanjay.kapil@okstate.edu (S. Kapil).

0195-5616/08/$ – see front matter
doi:10.1016/j.cvsm.2008.02.009

Published by Elsevier Inc.
vetsmall.theclinics.com

or dogs whenever they are brought into situations in which groups of animals are housed together, even temporarily, such as at greyhound racetracks, kennels, catteries, animal shelters, animal obedience training classes, dog parks, pet stores, pet day care facilities. This is especially true when pets are allowed by their owners to roam at will, commingling with ownerless feral dogs and cats and wildlife. For example, the rapid spread of CPV-2, which is extremely stable in the environment and highly contagious, was caused not only by the movement of dogs by their owners but by the transfer of fecal material on shoes and clothing of travelers and, unintentionally, through national and international mail [1].

According to the 2007 to 2008 National Pet Owners Survey conducted by the American Pet Products Manufacturers Association, the US pet cat population is estimated to be 88.3 million and the pet dog population is estimated to be 74.8 million [4]. Municipalities throughout the United States commonly pass animal control ordinances to protect the public health and safety and general welfare of the citizens and animals residing within the city. Typically, animal control codes limit the numbers of companion animals that individuals may own or keep on their private property, require that cats and dogs be licensed annually by owners and vaccinated against rabies, prevent animals from running at large, require proper disposal of animal waste, and prevent the feeding of wild or feral cats or dogs. Vaccination of dogs and cats by compliant pet owners for rabies prevention has, since 1960, dramatically reduced the occurrence of this disease; currently, most animal cases reported to the Centers for Disease Control and Prevention (CDC) now occur in wildlife [5]. Compliance with other animal control ordinances is variable, particularly among pet owners with respect to leash laws for dogs and cats and among well-intentioned individuals who maintain wild or feral colonies of cats and dogs by providing food, water, and shelter. Statistics from the Humane Society of the United States indicate that 6 to 8 million companion animals are admitted to shelters each year and nearly half are adopted or reclaimed by their owners, whereas the remaining animals are euthanized [6]. No census of ownerless dogs and cats is available. Estimates of the feral cat population in the United States range from 60 million to 100 million animals living primarily in or near urban settings with ample opportunity to interact with pets that are allowed to roam and with wildlife [7]. Thus, ownerless, wild, or feral dog and cat populations may transmit infectious and zoonotic diseases between wildlife and companion animals. From a public health standpoint, this is of particular importance because emerging viral infections from wildlife are often transmitted to human beings by means of a pet that is allowed to stray.

It is widely believed by virologists and public health epidemiologists that most viruses emerging from wildlife have an RNA or single-strand DNA genome [8] because they have a high propensity for mutation. Two significant canine viruses have emerged recently and meet this hypothesis: CPV and canine distemper virus (CDV). Canine distemper has re-emerged in the past decade [9,10] because of antigenic and genetic drift in the surface protein (H glycoprotein). In a multicontinent study, variant CDV strains, (but not the vaccine strain of CDV virus) were the cause of illness within 2 weeks after vaccination. In 2005 and 2006, large outbreaks of CPV variants (CPV-2c and CPV-2b*) in kennels occurred in Oklahoma and other states [10]. Diagnostic and molecular studies detected mutations in the parvovirus isolates that explained the failures of current commercial CPV vaccines from conferring protection and of approved commercial diagnostic kits from detecting these new viral isolates. Another recent example is outbreaks of hemorrhagic symptoms associated with virulent feline calicivirus (FCV) in the United States [11]; however, molecular basis of gain of virulence in FCV is not yet understood. In addition to virus evolution, in some cases, the virus can be reintroduced back after the population immunity has declined after a period of disease-free status. Thus, diseases that have been eradicated from developed countries but are still circulating in developing countries [12] may re-emerge by reintroduction from trade or movement of animals.

There is a major commitment by the US Department of Agriculture (USDA) in this country and in cooperation with foreign governments and international agencies worldwide to monitor the health of food animals and certain wildlife but not of companion animals [13]. The primary mission of the CDC is to promote and protect human health. To this end, the CDC performs surveillance for noninfectious and infectious diseases, including zoonoses [14]; however, the only chosen reportable viral diseases of animals that are collected by the CDC are rabies and avian influenza (H5N1), and those that are reported to the CDC ArboNET system are avian, animal, or mosquito WNV infections. Largely, surveillance of companion animal diseases, many of which have zoonotic potential, has not been considered to be a priority until recently [15,16]. In 2004, the CDC partnered with the Purdue University School of Veterinary Medicine to establish a pilot surveillance system to monitor clinical syndromes and diseases of small animals [17] to determine whether animals can serve as sentinels of health hazards to human beings. The National Companion Animal Surveillance Program (NCASP) initially drew exclusively on the database of the privately owned organization, Banfield, the Pet Hospital, which provides medical care to approximately 1.6 million pet dogs and cats in 44 states, and it now integrates data from Antech Diagnostics to detect potential emerging and zoonotic infections. A long-term goal of the NCASP is to become a national resource in veterinary public health. In the meantime, the front line of companion animal surveillance for emerging diseases is at the home front, with astute small animal clinicians playing a major role.

It can be a challenge for busy and isolated veterinary practices to receive the information on emerging viruses. Linking to a health-related network for companion animals might fill the gap. Recently, a space-time permutation scan statistic, which was applied in the anthrax terrorist attacks in 2001 [18], WNV outbreaks [19], and enzootic raccoon rabies [20], has been applied to veterinary diagnostic data in the Unite States and Europe [21]. This analysis provides important information about potential clusters of medical conditions and issues medical alerts about the developing situations based on mortality and confirmed diagnosis of important disease conditions. Earlier and more timely notifications should lead to more thorough investigations and reduce losses, especially from emerging viral diseases. It is important to keep in mind that clinical syndromes tend to be multifactorial, and it is essential to review the entire history, including environmental factors, with the specialist in a small animal specialty practice and also with a small animal teaching hospital before arriving at a conclusion about the case.

The purpose of this article is to encourage companion animal veterinarians to think outside the routine diagnostic plan when atypical cases of infectious disease are presented at their practices. Detecting emerging viral diseases of companion animals requires interaction and discussion among clinicians, pathologists, and virologists, and practicing small animal veterinarians must stay engaged in communication with these specialists through their state diagnostic laboratories or nearby colleges of veterinary medicine. Veterinary diagnostic medicine is rapidly progressing, and it is critical for the successful practitioner to stay abreast of new developments in small animal infectious diseases and their diagnosis through continuing education [22–24]. The development of monoclonal antibody technology in the 1980s and the advent of the polymerase chain reaction (PCR) assay in the 1990s have reshaped veterinary diagnostic strategies, especially in the subspecialty of virology. Now, these molecular techniques, which are becoming mainstream applications in routine viral diagnoses, are proving their merit in facilitating the diagnosis of emerging animal viruses. The authors offer practical information on the applications of diagnostic techniques for investigating viral disease outbreaks in companion animals. The authors provide this brief overview of diagnostic techniques in the modern virology laboratory that are used for routine diagnosis and in identifying novel and emerging viruses. Every step of diagnostic investigation—history, specimen collection, transportation, and laboratory examination—has to be carefully aligned for optimal outcome.

CLINICAL HISTORY AND SPECIMEN COLLECTION
Clinical History
Small animal clinicians are familiar with symptoms of common infectious diseases and are often the first to recognize the emergence of new disease problems. In some cases, there may be a history of vaccination compliance, yet some animals develop disease [25,26]. It is important to record the complete history, including the body system involved (eg, respiratory, gastrointestinal, reproductive tract, nervous system), clinical symptoms and their duration, the presence of lesions, and vaccination history. Particularly when the case is confounding, the client must be carefully and thoroughly interviewed as to how he or she manages the pet (ie, is the pet free to roam; has the pet traveled recently and where; if this is a new pet, where and how was it obtained; are there other pets in the household). Consulting a book on differential diagnoses can be useful to list the potential causes [27,28]. When a history of unusual symptoms is presented, clinicians, recognizing that these cases may be

important to individual and universal animal health, should refer these cases to an accredited veterinary diagnostic laboratory. It is convenient to attach copies of all relevant hospital records to the laboratory submission form to aid the diagnostician. Correct diagnosis depends on a thorough case history of the affected animal and submission of appropriate specimens that are collected and transported in a manner to preserve the integrity of the viral agent.

Specimen Collection

Submitting a comprehensive collection of specimens in a timely manner to the diagnostic laboratory from affected animals when the disease does not fit a familiar clinical picture, as is the case with emerging viral diseases, is of paramount importance. All the system(s) that are potentially involved and all the tissues with gross lesions should be sent to the diagnostic laboratory. It is important to check for concurrent infections. Viral diagnosis depends on the quality and type of specimen collected [29]. The best time for collection of specimens is immediately after symptoms of disease are first noticed. Samples from all body systems involved in the acute stage of the disease of affected animals should be submitted to the diagnostic laboratory in a timely manner by overnight delivery. At least 1 to 5 g or mL of each sample should be collected. Recovery of virus in cell culture depends on the condition of the specimen received by the diagnostic laboratory. Freezing specimens can be detrimental to virus isolation efforts (and also to electron microscopic identification) and should only be done ($-70°C$) if it is not possible to deliver the specimen to the laboratory within 48 hours. Use wet ice for shipping virology samples, because dry ice (solid carbon dioxide gas) can inactivate many viruses, preventing isolation in cell culture. Tissues intended for virus isolation should always be shipped in separate packages from specimens that are immersed in formalin to prevent fumes of formaldehyde from reaching the fresh tissues.

It is imperative that tissues and organs from animals that have died be harvested as soon as possible after death. Postmortem tissues should be placed in sterile containers with a small amount of transport medium (1–2 mL), if possible. When the clinician is unsure as to what specific organs and fluids should be retrieved, the entire carcass of the dog or cat may be delivered to the laboratory for examination. To obtain more specific details regarding specimen collection, packaging, and submission, contact the diagnostic laboratory of your choice by telephone or consult its specimen submission and fee schedule guidelines, which are often available on an Internet Web site.

Individuals who ship biologic substances for diagnostic testing are required by federal law to be in compliance with all regulations governing packaging and labeling of interstate shipments of causative agents. Failure to follow the regulations results in heavy fines (Fig. 1). Complete instructions on appropriate packaging for laboratory specimens to be mailed or shipped by a common carrier may be accessed in several sections of the Code of Federal Regulations (CFR). Health and Human Service regulations define such terms as *diagnostic specimen* and *etiologic agent* and describe requirements for packaging and labeling

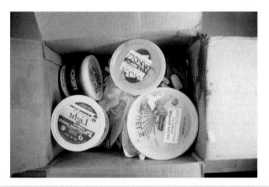

Fig. 1. Improper packaging of clinical samples. This submission is unsuitable because no ice packs were used. Instead, Styrofoam peanuts were added with wooden shavings. These packing materials can be a source of contamination and do not provide any advantage. Recycled food containers are unsuitable because they are a source of food microorganisms.

of these materials for shipping in Title 42 CFR Part 72. Department of Transportation regulations for shipping and packaging are found in Title 49 CFR Part 173, including definitions of infectious substances (49 CFR 173.134) and requirements concerning shipments containing dry ice (49 CFR 173.217). Regulations for airline shipments of dangerous goods are also available through the International Air Transport Association (IATA) [30]. The US Postal Service and most commercial delivery services (eg, United Parcel Service [UPS]; Federal Express [FedEx]; and Dalsey, Hillblom, Lynn [DHL]) provide packing information on request.

LABORATORY METHODS

Viruses have a simple structure with a protein coat enclosed with only one type of nucleic acid (DNA or RNA) rather than both. Thus, methods for viral diagnosis target one of the components of the virus structure. For a definitive viral disease diagnosis, four basic approaches are used: direct detection by virus isolation or direct identification, viral serology for detection of a specific antibody, viral antigen detection, and molecular-based detection of genetic material. A brief discussion of the principles of diagnostic assays representative of each approach follows.

Gross Pathologic and Histopathologic Findings

Histologic (Fig. 2) and cytologic examination (Fig. 3) of tissues and fluids by a board-certified veterinary pathologist contributes valuable information about the pathologic signs, gross and microscopic, that distinguish infections caused by viral or bacterial pathogens and other possible etiologies. Tissue tropism, mononuclear infiltrates, development of inclusion bodies (intranuclear, cytoplasmic, or both), and the formation of syncytia are some of the characteristics that differ among viruses and can sometimes distinguish different viral infections. For example, most DNA viruses replicate in the nucleus, and thus

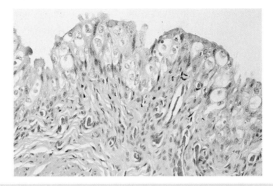

Fig. 2. Section of bladder from a dog with CDV. Eosinophilic inclusion bodies are present in the bladder epithelium. (*Courtesy of* Gregory Campbell, DVM, MS, PhD, Stillwater, OK.)

tend to produce intranuclear inclusions, whereas most RNA viruses form cytoplasmic inclusions, although there are exceptions. As part of the pathologist's examination, immunohistochemistry testing (Figs. 4 and 5), fluorescent antibody testing, and possibly in situ hybridization (ISH) studies on tissues may be ordered; these methods are considered elsewhere in this article. A complete histopathology report should include possible differentials for the lesions. The pathologist might note that some findings do not exactly fit the routine lesions he or she has observed in previously. In cases in which there are deviations in lesion type or distribution or when gross lesions and histopathologic findings

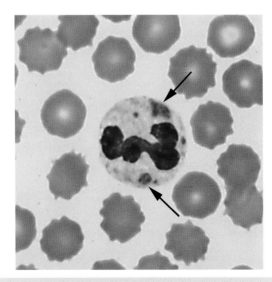

Fig. 3. Blood smear stained with aqueous Romanowsky stain shows intracytoplasmic inclusion bodies (*arrows*) confirmed to be positive for CDV.

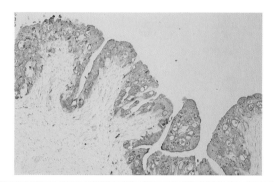

Fig. 4. Immunoperoxidase staining for CDV in the bladder of a dog. (*Courtesy of* Gregory Campbell, DVM, MS, PhD, Stillwater, OK.)

suggest the involvement of a viral disease but routine virology tests do not detect the expected conventional viral agents, variant or "emerging" viruses or even iatrogenic infections may be suspected. In early 1990, blue tongue virus serotype 11 was introduced in canine populations from a commercial modified-live multivalent canine vaccine that was associated with high mortality in dogs [31,32]. In some situations, second or even third opinions from pathologists at other laboratories who have special expertise should be solicited [33]. With the application of telepathology to veterinary case materials, networks of specialists, including veterinary pathologists, small animal clinicians, infectious disease specialists, and laboratory diagnosticians, are able to exchange patient histories, clinical data, and images (gross and microscopic) through the Internet for consultation, diagnosis, and education. This allows timely access to expert opinions at other locations throughout the world [34,35]. The use of telepathology can facilitate rapid intervention through the synergy of

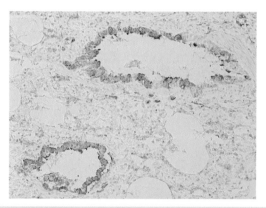

Fig. 5. Immunoperoxidase staining of a section of lung. The bronchiolar epithelium is positive for CDV antigen. (*Courtesy of* Gregory Campbell, DVM, MS, PhD, Stillwater, OK.)

computer technology and special pathology expertise (eg, system- and species-specific pathologic findings) to understand the lesions in difficult cases better.

DIRECT DETECTION

Virus Isolation

Conventional virus isolation techniques are often the backbone of investigation of novel viral diseases, provided that the virus is cultivable in available cell lines or primary cell cultures. Virus isolation may be relatively slow depending on the growth characteristics of the virus; however, roller culturing or centrifugation of samples onto cell monolayer(s) can enhance viral replication and recovery. In many of the recent emerging viruses from wildlife (eg, bats), the virus was first cultivated, allowing further characterization of the virus. It is important to keep in mind that virus isolation, even if the effort is successful, may have a slow turn-around time, approximately 2 to 3 weeks. Definitive identification of virus in cell culture can only be accomplished with specific antibody nucleic acid testing, and in the case of an "emerging" virus, existing reagents may not be reactive with the "new" virus. If culture is successful, however, the viral material may be studied by electron microscopy (EM) and by molecular techniques, as described in this article, to characterize the new isolate. Virus isolation requires fresh tissues and cannot be done on formalin-fixed tissues.

Physical and Chemical Methods That Aid in Identification of Viruses

EM is often used in veterinary diagnostic laboratories to detect enteric viruses in fecal samples retrieved during the course of viral diarrheal disease. Additionally, EM is indispensable for identification of emerging and previously unidentified viruses in clinical samples [36], and this method has helped in the identification of many new viruses, including, most recently, bat Lyssavirus [37]. Viruses can be classified up to the virus family based on size, shape, and distinctive structural features, such as envelopes or protein spikes, particularly for parvovirus, rotavirus (Fig. 6), coronavirus, astrovirus, herpesvirus,

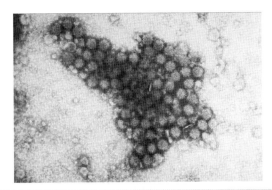

Fig. 6. Detection of rotavirus particles by EM. Most virus particles are similar in size and shape. The picture shows a few empty rotavirus particles.

poxvirus, and picornavirus. EM allows detection of multiple viruses simulta-neously. Application of antibodies to supplement the EM diagnosis provides higher sensitivity and further confirmation of the viral diagnosis. Sensitivity is the major limitation of EM, and at least 10^5 to 10^7 virus particles per milliliter must be present in the sample being examined. Because the electron micro-scope is an expensive piece of equipment that requires special technical skills and a high level of expertise, it is not available in many laboratories. Viral com-ponents can also be determined by several basic biochemistry experiments.

Acridine orange (AO) staining can determine the nature of the nucleic acid of purified viral particles [38]. Differentiation as to whether the nucleic acid is sin-gle- or double-stranded in nature is based on the color developed on AO stain-ing; double-stranded DNA or RNA nucleic acids stain yellow green, whereas single-stranded DNA or RNA acids stain flame red. Nuclease susceptibility of the purified virions differentiates DNA from RNA. The presence of enve-lope on viruses can be determined by susceptibility to the virus to heat, ether, or other lipid solvents [39]. The titrated virus preparation is treated with ether or chloroform. A decrease in virus titer of greater than 1 log is considered to be significant to indicate the presence of envelope on the virus. The presence of envelope indicates that virus is susceptible to common disinfectants. Lack of envelope indicates that the virus is resistant to the use of common disinfectants.

ANTIBODY DETECTION METHODS
Serology
Classic serology tests indirectly determine the viral etiology of disease by detecting the presence of antibody in serum (red-topped tube) to a specific test viral antigen, and thus provide retrospective evidence of an immune re-sponse or exposure to a virus. Serologic methods still provide powerful tools in the virology laboratory of today for diagnosing viral diseases that are seen routinely and for discovering and characterizing novel viral diseases. Serologic tests are now used to detect antibody or antigen in serum and body fluids. Typ-ically, methods used in the virology laboratory are serum neutralization (SN), hemagglutination-inhibition (HAI) test, indirect fluorescent antibody test (IFAT), and ELISA. Serologic results require interpretation by an expert diag-nostician based on critical clinical observations, confirmation by pathology ex-amination, virus isolation, and mass screening of the populations by serology. If animals in populations that have never been exposed to or vaccinated against a given virus have specific antibodies detected in their serum, it is expected that this is most likely attributable to recent exposure to the emerging virus. Paired serum samples are important to demonstrate a fourfold significant increase in antibody titers, which indicates that the diagnosis of recent exposure may be attributable to infection as opposed to previous exposure or vaccination depending on the vaccination history. Serology is also useful to study the antigenic distance of the emerging virus and provides clues as to whether the newly emerged agent is or is not likely to be protected by an available vac-cine(s), such as heterologous virus in another species of animal.

Hemagglutination Inhibition

Viral hemagglutination (HA) occurs between the viral protein; hemagglutinin (HN), which is present on the viral capsid or envelope of only certain families of viruses; and specific receptors on red blood cells (RBCs) that bind to HN, causing their agglutination and precipitation from solution. This phenomenon is the basis for a powerful and sensitive assay, the HAI test. When a hemagglutinating virus is mixed with serum containing antibodies specific to that virus, RBCs that are added to the mixture do not agglutinate and precipitate from solution. Feline panleukopenia, CPV, influenza A, and parainfluenza antibodies may be detected by HAI testing. The HAI method may also be used to identify unknown virus utilizing antibodies of known specificity; however, most often, this test is applied to detect the presence of antibodies in a serum sample against specific hemagglutinating viruses. Variants of CPV and feline parvovirus can differ in the hemagglutinating activity of swine erythrocytes [40,41].

Serum Neutralization

SN measures the inhibitory activity of a hyperimmune serum against viral isolates in cell culture. Commonly performed in a cell culture microwell format, this is a long-standing method for quantifying virus-specific antibodies, and it is usually performed to test for antibodies to viruses that typically cause cell damage (cytopathic effect [CPE]) to the host cell culture they infect. When a virus is mixed with hyperimmune serum containing antibodies specific to that virus, the antibodies bind the virus, preventing infection of the cell culture. The SN test can diagnose current infection using acute and convalescent serum samples from individual animals. It may also be used to determine immune status conferred on vaccinated animals. Vaccination antibody titers often differ from antibody titers developed in response to natural infection. Usually, vaccination titers are lower relative to infection titers, and maximal titers occur approximately 21 to 30 days after vaccination. SN assays are commonly performed to detect antibodies to FCV, herpesvirus, enteric coronavirus, and syncytial viruses and to canine herpesvirus, CDV, coronavirus, parainfluenza virus, and adenovirus.

ELISA

This is useful for screening large numbers of samples for the presence of antibodies against viruses. The ELISA format is flexible, and it may be used to detect antibody or antigen in clinical specimens. In either case, the detection system is an antibody conjugated to an enzyme. When the enzyme-linked antibody binds to the analyte being measured, the enzyme reacts with a chromogenic substrate, causing a color change to occur that may be measured spectrophotometrically or evaluated visually. Several ELISA kits are available to detect antiviral antibodies in companion animals, including CPV and CDV, feline leukemia virus (FeLV), feline immunodeficiency virus (FIV), and feline coronavirus. The immunoglobulin M (IgM) ELISA is a method used to distinguish current infection from past infection. During acute disease or immediately after vaccination with modified-live viruses, IgM is the first class of

KAPIL, YEARY, & JOHNSON

immunoglobulin produced in response to infection, appearing 1 to 2 weeks before there are detectable levels of IgG in the serum. Because it is short-lived, IgM levels typically disappear 3 months after infection. A single acute-phase serum test sample is sufficient to diagnose current infection with an IgM ELISA. Testing of IgM titers is available for several viral agents, including CDV and CPV among others. ELISA is useful for screening naive animal populations for the presence of antibodies against viruses to track the origin and spread of emerging infections. Antibodies to WNV have recently been detected in dogs and cats by IgM-capture ELISA [42]. A related method known as virus neutralization can be used to identify the serotype of a newly discovered virus.

Western Blot Assay (Immunoblot Assay)

Western blot (WB) may be used as a supplementary test to confirm antibody ELISA results for FIV testing [43]. To perform the assay, purified virus is disrupted using detergent; the constituent proteins are then separated on the basis of molecular weight by electrophoresis in a polyacrylamide gel. The proteins are transferred (blotted) from the gel to a nitrocellulose or polytetrafluoroethylene (PTFE) membrane for stabilization. The electrophoretically separated proteins are the antigen substrates for analyzing the test sera for the presence of specific antibodies. As with the ELISA format, the Western immunoblot uses an enzyme-labeled antispecies antibody that binds to the test serum antibodies that have bound to the separated viral antigens. Substrate reacting with the enzyme-labeled antibody in the presence of a colorless soluble benzidine derivative results in conversion to colored insoluble precipitate at the protein bands where test serum antibodies are bound. The molecular weight of the protein detected is characteristic for a particular viral component. Immunoblot results of the unknown test antisera are compared with positive control test sera for interpretation. A major advantage of the immunoblot technique is that a full antibody profile of a single serum sample is made simultaneously, identifying each of the individual particulate viral antigens that patient antibodies bind. As an epidemiologic tool, WB analysis may be used to detect currently circulating viral subtypes within a population and to characterize new emerging viral subtypes. Immunoblotting is also a valuable research technique for antigen detection that is often used to characterize novel viruses by comparing them with known related viral family members using standard antisera or monoclonal antibodies.

ANTIGEN DETECTION METHODS

Immunofluorescence Assays

Immunofluorescence assays on cells from clinical samples can be applied for rapid diagnostic investigations (30–45 minutes), provided that the fluorescent microscope and expertise are available in a laboratory. With the pooling of primary monoclonal antibodies against potential viral agents, the assay can be used as a screening tool and the sample tested again with individual conjugates to obtain specific virus diagnosis (Fig. 7).

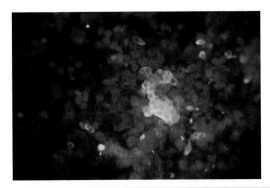

Fig. 7. Direct fluorescent antibody test. Cells show intracytoplasmic staining for coronavirus multiplying in the nasal cells. The negative cells stain brick red. The positive cells stain apple green.

ELISA for Antigen Detection

The ELISA is also a means for detecting viral antigens present in clinical specimens, and it offers a relatively quick turn-around time. Antigen test ELISA kits are available to detect antiviral antigens in companion animals, including CPV, FeLV, and FIV. Additionally, it is a common practice by many veterinary diagnostic laboratories to appropriate the use of some rapid antigen test kits intended for the human diagnostic market, specifically, rotavirus test kits. When monoclonal antibodies are used as capture antibodies in ELISA test kits, however, they fail if there is a mutation in the epitope of the viral surface protein present in the specimen that is being tested. Lateral flow immunoassay is a special application of the ELISA that provides a rapid, economic, portable, sensitive, and specific technique that is convenient for performing testing outside of the laboratory. It is the technique of choice for emerging viral infections [44,45], and it has gained attention for use in diagnosing foreign animal diseases and zoonotic and emerging viral infections of animals, such as influenza virus and WNV, in the field. The test kits are small in size (size of credit cards), extremely stable at ambient temperature (25°C), and take minutes to perform.

MOLECULAR-BASED METHODS

An advantage of nucleic acid–based testing is that specimens submitted for analysis do not have to have viable viral particles present to be detected by this means. There is a trend toward application of molecular or gene sequence–based techniques to routine virology testing in diagnostic laboratories, which is justified under several circumstances. First, a molecular technique may be the test of choice if conventional methods of diagnosis are technically weak, such as when a viral agent is noncultivable or there are biocontainment concerns with culturing the virus, the virus has amorphous morphology by EM, antibodies are unavailable or not specific to the virus, and serologic tests result in a confounding diagnosis. Second, molecular techniques may be essential to detect and classify the sequence type or genotype of a virus. Third, a viral agent may be characteristically slow to replicate, such as γ-herpes virus; thus, a molecular method might provide a better turn-around time for diagnosis. In this instance, a rapid diagnosis might be achieved by pan-herpesvirus PCR. Finally, a novel viral isolate that cannot be definitively identified by the routine diagnostic methods described previously may merit investigation and characterization by molecular-based techniques, which are indispensable in the classification of new and emerging viruses. These advanced techniques may confirm a diagnosis of viral etiology when other tests have failed; however, they are, unfortunately, relatively expensive. Furthermore, the presence of nucleic acid does not equate to infection, and infections are attributable to subclinical, latency-associated nucleic acids or defective interfering virus particles, such as in paramyxoviruses, produced in nonproductive infections in genetically resistant hosts. Clients, who bear the financial burden, should be counseled as to the benefit and shortfalls of this testing before ordering molecular-based tests. An excellent review of molecular-based techniques for diagnostic testing of infectious diseases has appeared in a previous issue in this series [46].

Polymerase Chain Reaction

The most familiar nucleic acid testing technique, PCR, has been used for more than a decade; however, over the past few years, real-time PCR has taken its place, revolutionizing diagnostic virology. In this procedure, the PCR chemistry may be combined with detection using a single-stranded DNA probe with a fluorescent label [47]. Moreover, the procedure may be completed within an hour, and it allows for quantitation of results. Because the hands-on steps are reduced and the PCR reactions are not opened, it eliminates the chances of cross-contamination in the laboratory. Real-time PCR protocols are gaining more acceptance in routine veterinary diagnosis.

In Situ Hybridization

ISH involves using nucleotide probes with an attached label. Non–isotope-labeled probes (digoxigenin or fluochrome) can be applied in veterinary diagnostic laboratories. Diagnostic applications of ISH involve identification of virus-specific sequences (DNA or RNA) in the tissues or cells [48]. Although uncommon in veterinary diagnostic laboratories, ISH is in routine use in human diagnostic laboratories for detection of the genotype of human papilloma viruses in cervical samples. For ISH, smears and tissues (fresh, unfrozen, and fixed tissues) are suitable.

Electropherotyping and Restriction Fragment Length Polymorphism

In electropherotyping and restriction fragment length polymorphism (RFLP), double-stranded DNA (RFLP) or RNA (electropherotypes) is purified and size-separated on agarose or acrylamide gel electrophoresis. Because nucleic acids are charged and double-stranded molecules bind more ethidium bromide compared with single-stranded nucleic acids, under the electric field, the nucleic acids migrate and larger sized molecules separate out higher than smaller sized molecules. For DNA molecules to be tested, the double-stranded viral DNA- or PCR-amplified fragments are digested with restriction enzymes. These techniques allow quick differentiation of viral genomes (DNA or RNA). Both techniques have applications in molecular epidemiology of rotaviruses [49].

NEW GENERATION MOLECULAR TECHNIQUES

Viral Genome Sequencing Technologies

Viral genome or mRNA sequencing is a powerful molecular epidemiologic tool and has been applied for epidemiology of rabies virus [50]. Sequences of novel or emerging viruses may be derived based on known conserved sequences of previously characterized viruses within the same family. Although virus sequencing is gaining more routine application in veterinary laboratories, it does add cost, and thus should be used judiciously. When these methods fail to identify a newly discovered virus, which is truly novel, metagenomic analysis, which is largely used in research laboratories, may be applied. Pyrosequencing is a recent variation on sequencing short stretches of PCR-generated DNA without the need for labeled primers, labeled nucleotides, and gel electrophoresis [51]. Although this variation on PCR and nucleic acid sequencing is currently used exclusively as a research tool, it is likely to be adapted for clinical diagnostic work in future years because it has been demonstrated to detect many different unrelated viruses simultaneously in a single reaction and to identify viral serotypes and detect viral isolates that could not previously be typed by classic procedures [52,53].

Microarray Platform

A biochip or microarray is small solid support, such as a nylon membrane, silicon chip, or glass slide, on which nucleic acid fragments, antibodies, or proteins are immobilized in an orderly arrangement. Thousands of different molecules, referred to as probes, may be machine-printed as spots on the support, allowing for high throughput of samples using lower volumes of analyte in less time than conventional laboratory techniques take to complete. Microarrays are essentially miniaturized laboratories that can perform hundreds or thousands of simultaneous biochemical reactions that are most commonly detected through the use of fluorophores. The fluorescent signal patterns formed by each analyte are then compared by the computer software using complex algorithms to make an identification of its contents. Biochips enable researchers to screen large numbers of biologic analytes quickly for a variety of purposes, ranging from disease diagnosis to detection of bioterrorism agents. Biochip technology is still relatively new and has not yet entered the mainstream of clinical diagnostics techniques, although it is widely used in research institutions. As an epidemiologic tool, the use of nucleic acid microarrays was instrumental in the rapid identification of the first severe acute respiratory syndrome (SARS) coronavirus outbreak in China [54]. Coronavirus protein microarrays have been used to screen Canadian sera [55] for specific antibodies to SARS and to other coronaviruses in a comparative study with the traditional ELISA.

Scientists around the world are assessing the feasibility of using microarrays as tools for surveillance and diagnosis of influenza viruses [56,57]. Once issues of sensitivity and assay validation have been addressed satisfactorily and the cost of the technology has become more affordable, microarray technology may find a place in clinical diagnosis.

ESTABLISHING VIRAL DISEASE CAUSATION

Pathogenic Virus or "Orphan" Virus or "Vaccine-Source" Virus

Molecular methods for detecting and identifying viral pathogens are powerful. It is possible to detect a virus in a specimen, but it may have no association with the clinical condition. These types of viruses are called "orphan viruses." Minute virus of canine is a parvovirus, and it causes no clinical disease [58]. As a result of the advent of sensitive molecular techniques, it is quite common to detect viral sequences of agents that may be present in a sample but not associated with the disease (orphan viral agents). It is possible to study the association of the viral agent with the pathologic findings observed to support the diagnosis. Moreover, the PCR protocols targeting structural genes that are expressed only during active infection are useful and avoid the potential false-positive results attributable to latency or persistent viral infections. Moreover, the sense and antisense probes offer the opportunity for resident and replication intermediates of viruses. Obviously, the history of recent vaccination should be known, and the vaccine virus from the same lot of vaccine should be simultaneously included in the testing run and sequenced over critical regions to ensure that the virus in the sample is the same or different from the vaccine.

Failure or Lack of Correlation Between Diagnostic Techniques

When fluorescent antibody testing or immunohistochemistry testing is performed, false-negative findings result even when a related virus is present. Because of changes in the sequence of the target protein epitopes, antibody-based detection methods may fail to provide the diagnosis; monoclonal antibodies used may fail to react and polyclonal antibodies may cross-react weakly when a variant strain of virus is present. Thus, a sudden trend in lack of correlation between tests may signal an emerging variant of the virus. If a new variant of the virus arises, it may be associated with a change in the clinical profile and we may or may not understand the molecular basis of this shift. It is possible that the polyclonal antibodies may react weakly with the new variant of the virus. In many cases, the PCR primers may fail to amplify the new variant if the mutation occurs in the hypervariable region of the target gene amplified. For example, in the recent emergence of CPV variants, many practitioners noted clinical symptoms compatible with CPV but the commercial field tests were not working. If a new variant of virus emerges, a polyclonal antibody antiserum prepared in a heterologous species (rabbit or goat) can be used as a primary antibody against the whole virus, because it is possible that the monoclonal antibody might fail. The molecular techniques are more likely to fail compared with the antibody-based techniques because of the degeneracy of codons. It is important to keep in mind that factors other than emerging viruses can also affect the performance of USDA-approved tests. For example, local anesthetic can also affect the outcome of antibody tests. In one study, the use of lidocaine was recommended over oxybuprocaine to avoid false-positive results [59].

SUMMARY

It should be clear to the readers that veterinarians are bound to encounter emerging viruses in their practice. The problem is unavoidable because viruses are "perfect" obligate parasites. Even the immune response dictates the nature of virus that evolves in a host. Thus, vaccines are to be viewed as preventive tools rather than as a cure for emerging viruses. In some situations, the best vaccine is bound to fail. Similarly, the diagnostic methods have to be tailor-fitted to keep up with the emerging viruses. If the clinical signs and diagnostic methods fail to correlate, the veterinarian should work with diagnostic laboratory to solve the diagnostic puzzle. Your state veterinary diagnostic laboratory may be the first place that issues an alert to veterinary professionals and the public at large to possible emerging viral diseases. Newsletters from your state diagnostic laboratory can be a good source of information about emerging viral diseases in your area. Additional sources that are dedicated to dog and cat health issues and public health are available on the Internet [60–68].

References

[1] Carmichael LE. An annotated historical account of canine parvovirus. J Vet Med B Infect Dis Vet Public Health 2005;52(7–8):303–11.

[2] Buonavoglia C, Martella V, Pratelli A, et al. Evidence for evolution of canine parvovirus type 2 in Italy. J Gen Virol 2001;82(12):3021–5.

[3] Kapil S, Cooper E, Lamm C, et al. Canine parvovirus types 2c and 2b circulating in North American dogs in 2006 and 2007. J Clin Microbiol 2007;45(12):4044–7.

[4] American Pet Products Manufacturers Association. Industry statistics and trends: 2007–2008 National Pet Owners Survey. Greenwich (CT): APPMA; Available at: http://www.appma.org/press_industrytrends.asp. Accessed March, 2008.

[5] Blanton JD, Hanlon CA, Rupprecht CE. Rabies surveillance in the United States during 2006. J Am Vet Med Assoc 2007;231(4):540–56.

[6] Humane Society of the United States. Available at: http://www.hsus.org/pets/. Accessed March, 2008.

[7] Stray Pet Advocacy. Feral cat population statistic. Available at: http://www.StrayPetAdvocacy.org. Accessed March, 2008.

[8] Parrish CR, Kawaoka Y. The origins of new pandemic viruses: the acquisition of new host ranges by canine parvovirus and influenza A viruses. Annu Rev Microbiol 2005;59:553–86.

[9] Decaro N, Campolo M, Lorusso A, et al. Experimental infection of dogs with a novel strain of canine coronavirus causing systemic disease and lymphopenia. Vet Microbiol 2008;128:253–60.

[10] Kapil S, Allison RW, Johnston L, et al. Canine distemper viruses circulating in North American dogs. Clin Vaccine Immunol 2008;15(4):707–12.

[11] Pedersen NC, Elliott JB, Glasgow A, et al. An isolated epizootic of hemorrhagic-like fever in cats caused by a novel and highly virulent strain of feline calicivirus. Vet Microbiol 2000;73(4):281–300.

[12] Rweyemamu MM. Future risks from infectious diseases of animals. Presented at the World Association of Veterinary Laboratory Diagnosticians, 13th International Symposium. Melbourne, Australia: 2007. p. 25.

[13] Lynn T, Marano N, Treadwell T, et al. Linking human and animal health surveillance for emerging diseases in the United States—achievements and challenges. Ann N Y Acad Sci 2006;1081:108–11.

[14] CDC Functional Mission Statement. United States Department of Health and Human Services Centers for Disease Control and Prevention. Available at: http://www.cdc.gov/about. Accessed March, 2008.

[15] National Research Council, Commission on Life Sciences, Board on Environmental Studies and Toxicology, et al. Animals as sentinels of environmental health hazards. Washington, DC: National Academy Press; 1991.

[16] World Health Organization. Future trends in veterinary public health. WHO Technical Report Series 907. 2002. Available at: http://whqlibdoc.who.int/trs/WHO_TRS_907.pdf. Accessed March, 2008.

[17] Glickman LT, Moore GE, Glickman NW, et al. Purdue University-Banfield National Companion Animal Surveillance Program for emerging and zoonotic diseases. Vector Borne Zoonotic Dis 2006;6(1):14–23.

[18] Goldenberg A, Shmueli G, Caruana RA, et al. Early statistical detection of anthrax outbreaks by tracking over-the-counter medication sales. Proc Natl Acad Sci USA 2002;99(8):5237–40.

[19] Mostashari F, Kulldorff M, Hartman JJ, et al. Dead bird clustering: a potential early warning system for West Nile virus activity. Emerg Infect Dis 2003;9(6):641–6.

[20] Recuenco S, Eidson M, Kulldorff M, et al. Spatial and temporal patterns of enzootic raccoon rabies adjusted for multiple covariates. Int J Health Geogr 2007;6:14.

[21] Norstrom M, Pfeiffer DU, Jarp J. A space-time cluster investigation of an outbreak of acute respiratory disease in Norwegian cattle herds. Prev Vet Med 2000;47(1–2):107–19.

[22] Kennedy M. Methodology in diagnostic virology. Vet Clin North Am Exot Anim Pract 2005;8(1):7–26.

[23] Yeary TJ, Kapil S. A primer on diagnostic virology: specimen selection and serology. A primer of veterinary diagnostic laboratory testing. Compendium on Continuing Education for the Practicing Veterinarian 2004:646–58.

[24] Yeary TJ, Kapil S. A primer on diagnostic virology: direct and molecular-based detection of viral pathogens. A primer of veterinary diagnostic laboratory testing. Compendium on Continuing Education for the Practicing Veterinarian 2004:730–40.

[25] Amude AM, Alfieri AA, Alfieri AF. Antemortem diagnosis of CDV infection by RT-PCR in distemper dogs with neurological deficits without the typical clinical presentation. Vet Res Commun 2006;30(6):679–87.

[26] Amude AM, Alfieri AA, Alfieri AF. Clinicopathological findings in dogs with distemper encephalomyelitis presented without characteristic signs of the disease. Res Vet Sci 2007;82(3):416–22.

[27] Gough A. Differential diagnosis in small animal medicine. Oxford: Blackwell Publishing; 2007.

[28] Thompson MS. Small animal medical differential diagnosis. St. Louis (MO): Saunders Elsevier; 2007.

[29] Storch GA. Diagnostic virology. In: Knipe DM, Howley PM, editors. Fields' virology. 5th edition. Philadelphia: Wolters Kluwer; 2007. p. 566–7.

[30] Available at: http://www.iata.org/training/cargo/. Accessed March, 2008.

[31] Akita GY, Ianconescu M, MacLachlan NJ, et al. Bluetongue disease in dogs associated with contaminated vaccine. Vet Rec 1994;134(11):283–4.

[32] Kapil S, Krueger D, Schmidt SP. Iatrogenic infection of a pregnant dog with bluetongue virus, serotype 11. Presented at the 13th Annual Meeting of the American Society for Virology. Madison (WI), July, 1994.

[33] Willard MD, Jergens AE, Duncan RB, et al. Interobserver variation among histopathologic evaluations of intestinal tissues from dogs and cats. J Am Vet Med Assoc 2002;220(8): 1177–82.
[34] Robinson Y. Telepathology: its role in disease diagnosis in meat hygiene. Presented at the World Association of Veterinary Laboratory Diagnosticians 13th International Symposium. Melbourne, Australia: 2007. p. 78.
[35] Weinstein RS. Static image telepathology in perspective. Hum Pathol 1996;27(2):99–101.
[36] Bannert N, Laue M. Overview of electron microscopy and its role in infectious disease diagnosis. Presented at the World Association of Veterinary Laboratory Diagnosticians 13th International Symposium. Melbourne, Australia: 2007. p. 77.
[37] Hyatt AD. Diagnostic electron microscopy: historical review and future. Presented at the World Association of Veterinary Laboratory Diagnosticians 13th International Symposium. Melbourne, Australia: 2007. p. 76.
[38] Jamison RM, Mayor HD. Acridine orange staining of purified rat virus strain X14. J Bacteriol 1965;90(5):1486–8.
[39] Binn LN, Lazar EC, Eddy GA, et al. Recovery and characterization of a minute virus of canines. Infect Immun 1970;1(5):503–8.
[40] Parrish CR, Burtonboy G, Carmichael LE. Characterization of a nonhemagglutinating mutant of canine parvovirus. Virology 1988;163(1):230–2.
[41] Cavalli A, Bozzo G, Decaro N, et al. Characterization of a canine parvovirus strain isolated from an adult dog. New Microbiol 2001;24(3):239–42.
[42] Kile JC, Panella NA, Komar N, et al. Serologic survey of cats and dogs during an epidemic of West Nile virus infection in humans. J Am Vet Med Assoc 2005;226(8):1349–53.
[43] Egberink HF, Lutz H, Horzinek MC. Use of Western blot and radioimmunoprecipitation for diagnosis of feline leukemia and feline immunodeficiency virus infections. J Am Vet Med Assoc 1991;199(10):1339–42.
[44] Esfandiari J, Klingeborn B. A comparative study of a new rapid and one-step test for the detection of parvovirus in faeces from dogs, cats, and mink. J Vet Med B Infect Dis Vet Public Health 2000;47(2):145–53.
[45] Lee KN, Lee YJ, Kim JW, et al. Simple rapid, on-site detection for diagnosis of animal disease. Presented at the Abstracts of the 13th International Symposium. Melbourne, Australia: 2007. p. 71.
[46] Sellon RK. Update on molecular techniques for diagnostic testing of infectious disease. Vet Clin North Am Small Anim Pract 2003;33(4):677–93.
[47] Espy MJ, Uhl JR, Sloan LM, et al. Real-time PCR in clinical microbiology: applications for routine laboratory testing. Clin Microbiol Rev 2006;19(1):165–256.
[48] McNicol AM, Farquharson MA. In situ hybridization and its diagnostic applications in pathology. J Pathol 1997;182(3):250–61.
[49] Schroeder BA, Kalmakoff J, Holdaway D, et al. The isolation of rotavirus from calves, foals, dogs and cats in New Zealand. N Z Vet J 1983;31(7):114–6.
[50] Woldehiwet Z. Clinical laboratory advances in the detection of rabies virus. Clin Chim Acta 2005;351(1–2):49–63.
[51] Ronaghi M. Pyrosequencing sheds light on DNA sequencing. Genome Res 2001;11:3–11.
[52] Gharizadeh B, Oggionni M, Zheng B, et al. Type-specific multiple sequencing primers: a novel strategy for reliable and rapid genotyping of human papillomaviruses by pyrosequencing technology. J Mol Diagn 2005;7(2):198–205.
[53] Silva PA, Diedrich S, de Paula Cardoso DD, et al. Identification of enterovirus serotypes by pyrosequencing using multiple sequencing primers. J Virol Methods 2007;148: 260–4.
[54] Wang D, Coscoy L, Zylberberg M, et al. Micro-array-based detection and genotyping of viral pathogens. Proc Natl Acad Sci USA 2002;99(24):15687–92.
[55] Zhu H, Hu S, Jona G, et al. Severe acute respiratory syndrome diagnostics using a coronavirus protein microarray. Proc Natl Acad Sci USA 2006;103(11):4011–6.

[56] Mehlmann M, Bonner AB, Williams JV, et al. Comparison of the MChip to viral culture, reverse transcription-PCR, and the QuickVue influenza A+B test for rapid diagnosis of influenza. J Clin Microbiol 2007;45(4):1234–7.

[57] Quan PL, Palacios G, Jabado OJ, et al. Detection of respiratory viruses and subtype identification of influenza A viruses by GreeneChipResp oligonucleotide microarray. J Clin Microbiol 2007;45(8):2359–64.

[58] Carmichael LE, Schlafer DH, Hashimoto A. Minute virus of canines (MVC, canine parvovirus type-1): pathogenicity for pups and seroprevalence estimate. J Vet Diagn Invest 1994;6(2): 165–74.

[59] Hoshino T, Takanashi T, Okada M, et al. Oxybuprocaine induces a false-positive response in immunochromatographic SAS Adeno test. Ophthalmology 2002;109(4):808–9.

[60] American Association of Public Health Veterinarians. Available at: http://www.avma.org/. Accessed March, 2008.

[61] American Association of Veterinary Laboratory Diagnosticians. Available at: http://www.aavld.org. Accessed March, 2008.

[62] American Veterinary Medical Association. Available at: http://www.avma.org. Accessed March, 2008.

[63] CDC: Healthy pets healthy people. Available at: http://www.cdc.gov/healthypets/. Accessed March, 2008.

[64] CDC. MMWR Morb Mortal Wkly Rep. Available at: http://www.cdc.gov/mmwr/. Accessed March, 2008.

[65] Congress of Research Workers in Animal Diseases (CRWAD). Available at: http://www.cvmbs.colostate.edu/microbiology/crwad/. Accessed March, 2008.

[66] National Association of State Public Health Veterinarians. Available at: http://www.nasphv.org/. Accessed March, 2008.

[67] United States Animal Health Association. Available at: http://www.usaha.org. Accessed March, 2008.

[68] Code of Federal Regulations (search engine). Available at: http://www.gpoaccess.gov/cfr/index.html. Accessed March, 2008.

Vet Clin Small Anim 38 (2008) 775–786

VETERINARY CLINICS
SMALL ANIMAL PRACTICE

Molecular Virology of Feline Calicivirus

Patricia A. Pesavento, DVM, PhD[a],*,
Kyeong-Ok Chang, DVM, PhD[b],
John S.L. Parker, BVMS, PhD[c]

[a]Department of Pathology, Microbiology, and Immunology, School of Veterinary Medicine, University of California, Davis, One Shields Avenue, 4206 VM3A, Davis, CA 95616–5270, USA
[b]Diagnostic Medicine and Pathobiology, College of Veterinary Medicine, Kansas State University, 1800 Denison Avenue, K228 Mosier, Manhattan, KS 66506–5601, USA
[c]Department of Microbiology and Immunology, Baker Institute for Animal Health, College of Veterinary Medicine, Cornell University, Hungerford Hill Road, Ithaca, NY 14853, USA

*C*aliciviridae are small, nonenveloped, positive-stranded RNA viruses. There are four established genera in the calicivirus family (*Norovirus, Sapovirus, Lagovirus,* and *Vesivirus*) and a fifth proposed genus (*Nabovirus* or *Becovirus*) [1,2]. *Norovirus* and *Sapovirus* are the most common causes worldwide for nonbacterial gastrointestinal disease in human beings [3]. Members of the other genera can cause a broad spectrum of disease in many different animals. These include fatal highly contagious disease (eg, rabbit hemorrhagic disease virus) and infections in species other than their original host ("species-jumpers"; eg, San Miguel sea lion virus). Much of our understanding of the molecular biology of the caliciviruses has come from the study of the naturally occurring animal caliciviruses. In particular, many studies have focused on the molecular virology of feline calicivirus (FCV), which reflects its importance as a natural pathogen of cats and the ease with which it can be studied in the laboratory. There are excellent and recent reviews of the clinical disease, epidemiology, and pathogenesis of FCV [4,5]. This article updates the reader on the current status of clinical behavior and pathogenesis and reviews the molecular biology of the feline *Caliciviridae*.

EPIDEMIOLOGY

Although FCV is commonly thought of as a pathogen of the oral cavity and upper respiratory tract, it was originally isolated from the gastrointestinal tract of cats in New Zealand [6]. Subsequent reports established that FCV is ubiquitous in cat populations worldwide. Estimates of the prevalence of FCV in different

Some of the unpublished work reported was funded by the George Sydney and Phyllis Redman Miller Trust in cooperation with the Winn Feline Foundation and by the Cornell Feline Health Center.

Corresponding author. E-mail address: papesavento@ucdavis.edu (P.A. Pesavento).

populations are based on the detection of virus shed into the oral cavity using viral isolation or reverse transcriptase polymerase chain reaction (RT-PCR) to detect viral RNA. Prevalence rates of between 2% and 40% have been reported in population cross-sectional studies [7–10]. A recent longitudinal study that examined FCV prevalence at intervals in five catteries over 15 to 46 months found that with individual samplings, prevalence varied from 0% to 91% and that, overall, the average prevalence for the five colonies varied from as low as 6% to as high as 75% [11]. Maintenance of high viral prevalence in a dense population may be explained by long-term shedders (cats shedding a single isolate for up to 75 days have been identified Ref. [12]), sequential infections with multiple isolates, episodes of reinfection [13], or any combination of these factors.

FCV-related disease causes high morbidity and usually low mortality, with only occasional instances of more virulent disease. Over the past 10 years, however, there have been several reports of unusually virulent systemic (VS) FCV disease associated with high mortality [14–17]. These differences in the severity of FCV disease are perhaps not surprising, given that characteristic features of FCVs include high genetic variability, a capacity to persist in infected individuals, stability in the environment, and ubiquity in feline populations worldwide.

CLINICAL DISEASE

Many cats infected with FCV do not have overt clinical disease. These animals may be persistently infected or be infected with FCV isolates that cause mild or not easily detectable disease. In those cats showing acute signs of disease in natural or experimental infections, the most consistent clinical findings are fever and lingual or oral ulceration. FCV in natural and experimental disease can also cause upper respiratory signs (eg, sneezing, rhinitis, conjunctivitis). In general, however, epidemiologic studies that have identified FCV in natural outbreaks of upper respiratory tract (URT) disease have noted that disease is most likely to be in conjunction with multiple other pathogens [8,9,18] and that not all isolates used in experimental studies cause respiratory disease.

Over a span of 35 years, a diverse spectrum of less typical clinical disease has been attributed to infection with FCV [14,15,17,19–21]. Virulent "biotypes" of FCV are viruses associated with disease signs that diverge from the mild signs typically found in the field. The classification of individual FCV isolates as virulent is inappropriate unless the isolate in question has been experimentally shown to reproduce the disease syndrome reliably. The severity and range of disease signs associated with FCV infection depend on the route of exposure [22,23], the presence of concurrent disease(s) [24], and the age of the animal [25] and are also likely to be associated with viral dose and the immune status of the host, including vaccine status. Interestingly, a recent epidemiologic study of FCV in catteries in the United Kingdom found individual cats that were exposed to FCV for long periods but did not seem to become infected [11]. This finding indicates that some cats may acquire protective immunity or be genetically less susceptible. Because these factors can cause considerable variability in FCV disease presentation, and because it is possible that a single isolate can cause extraordinary disease in a particular animal, some FCV isolates have been categorized as virulent when, in fact, under other circumstances, they produce more typical FCV-related disease [22,23,25]. Therefore, even under experimental conditions, infection of specific pathogen free (SPF) cats with a single strain of virus can cause variable clinical outcomes. It has recently been demonstrated that the chronic carrier state is associated with emergence of antigenically, and perhaps biologically, distinct viruses [26]. These phenomena, along with variance in sequence generated in vitro (John S.L. Parker and Patricia A. Pesavento, unpublished data, 2004) before inoculation, could all contribute to the variability in morbidity, mortality, or clinical signs. At this point, a good number of virulent FCV isolates have been collected, and their associated clinical disease has been described. In nearly all cases, the atypical manifestations of disease occur together with the more common signs of FCV infection.

CLINICAL SYNDROMES ASSOCIATED WITH FELINE CALICIVIRUS INFECTION

"Limping Disease"

Three independent isolates of FCV (FCV2280, F65, and FCV-LLK) have been associated with "limping syndrome." Terwee and colleagues [23] and Dawson and colleagues [19] have reproduced limping by viral inoculation of SPF cats or kittens. In these studies, viruses were inoculated by multiple routes, with the most consistent clinical signs and histologic lesions (acute, severe, hemorrhagic, and neutrophilic synovitis) seen in joints inoculated directly with virus. Other routes of infection inconsistently caused synovitis or "limping disease." Limping or lameness has also been described in some cats naturally or experimentally infected with strains considered clinically to be associated exclusively with oral disease or respiratory disease [25] and in natural and experimental virulent systemic disease (VSD).

Lower Respiratory Tract Disease

Although mild URT infection associated with FCV is considered typical in a field situation, severe pneumonia is considered atypical. Isolates of FCV capable of causing severe bronchointerstitial pneumonia were among the first identified highly virulent isolates [27,28]. One experimental infection with pneumonic FCV included histologic and ultrastructural studies that demonstrated severe diffuse alveolar damage [29]. Although experimental reproduction of these identified "pneumonic isolates" is limited, there are multiple and recent reports of severe pneumonia with high mortality attributed to infection with FCV (Patricia A. Pesavento, unpublished data, 2005–2006).

Virulent Systemic Disease

Sporadically, over the past 10 years, FCV has been associated with outbreaks of severe systemic disease associated with high mortality. This syndrome was first recognized in 1998, and the disease was subsequently reproduced experimentally using calicivirus isolates collected from the field cases [15]. Initially, the disease was described as a "hemorrhagic-like fever." Because hemorrhage was not a consistent finding in subsequent but otherwise similar outbreaks, however, the disease has been renamed VSD and the associated FCV isolates are called virulent-systemic caliciviruses (VS-FCVs) [14,16]. *Virulent systemic disease* is a term used to describe a constellation of epidemiologic, clinical, and pathologic findings in affected cats. The clinical findings of VSD include fever nonresponsive to antibiotics and ulceration of the oral cavity (typically lingual, mucocutaneous junctions, and nose) and can include edema of the head, pinnae, and one or more paws; skin ulceration (eg, pinnae, footpads, lower extremities); jaundice; and an approximate mortality rate of 50%. Among the natural outbreaks that have been described [12,14,15,17], as many as 20 to 50 animals have been affected [12,17]; however, more typically, smaller numbers of animals are affected [14] (Patricia A. Pesavento, unpublished data, 2002–2007). A troubling feature of the disease is that in all the reported cases, vaccinated cats have been susceptible. In addition, a recent report described signs consistent with VSD in a captive tiger cub, adult African lions, and Amur tigers [30]. In this report, FCV RNA was detected in oral secretions and in multiple tissues from two of the affected animals that died during the outbreak.

VSD has been experimentally reproduced with four independent isolates of VS-FCV [15,31] (Patricia A. Pesavento, unpublished data, 2005 and 2008). Analysis of the genomic sequences has shown that VS-FCV isolates seem to have arisen independently from different genetic backgrounds, however [32]. As yet, no genetic signature has been identified that can discriminate VS-FCV isolates from other FCV isolates. Because of this and because FCV is highly prevalent in feline populations, it is difficult to establish definitively that FCV is the causative agent of VSD in natural outbreaks without isolating the virus and experimentally reproducing the disease. Thus, at present, FCV isolates recovered from cases with clinical and pathologic signs that fit a diagnosis of VSD should be presumptively characterized as VS-FCV. Despite their disparate genetic backgrounds, VS-FCV isolates seem to have a greater propensity to spread in tissue culture than non-VS isolates [32]. It is unclear if this in vitro phenomenon relates to their increased virulence, however.

Most systemic viral infections spread by means of the blood, and the degree and duration of viremia are likely important determinants of pathogenicity [33]. Although FCV has been isolated from the blood (P.A. Pesavento and others) of FCV-infected cats, the degree and duration of viremia have not been described for any experimental FCV infection. In the past, it was thought that viral spread during limited viral infections of epithelial tissues (as seen during most FCV infections) occurred by infection of contiguous tissues and that viremia did not occur or was uncommon. More recently, however, this paradigm has been challenged, and it is now thought that many viruses previously thought to be restricted to epithelial tissues have a viremic phase. Thus, one possible reason for the increased virulence of VS-FCV isolates might be an enhanced capacity to enter the bloodstream as free virus or in association with cells.

There are limited studies on tissue distribution of FCV. Published reports indicate that tissue tropism is expanded in VSD compared with non-VSD cases and that there is generally a correlation between tissue distribution and the development of lesions. All published reports describe viral protein distribution in one to two [14,34,35], or at most seven [16], cats from spontaneous outbreaks of disease, however. In non-VSD cases, viral protein detected by immunohistochemistry has been associated with the cytoplasm of skin epithelial cells [34,35], oral mucosa [36], and in macrophages isolated from joint fluid [37]. In spontaneous [14,16] and experimental (Patricia A. Pesavento, unpublished data, 2005) cases of VSD, viral protein, in addition to being detected in mucosal, skin, and respiratory epithelial cells, was variably found within pancreatic acinar cells, endothelial cells [16], and hepatocytes [14]. Distribution of virus was confirmed by ultrastructural studies in two reports of VSD [14,16].

Other Biotypes
Other disease syndromes occasionally associated with FCV are abortion [38] and neurologic signs (agitation) [21]. In both cases, although FCV was isolated from affected tissues, the disease was not reproduced experimentally. There is also a proposed association between FCV and chronic gingivitis or stomatitis [39,40]; however, the relation has been drawn by correlation of shedding with clinical signs, and in published attempts to reproduce this disease [24,41], none of the cats developed chronic stomatitis. The inability to reproduce chronic gingivitis or faucitis despite correlative evidence of FCV association indicates that other factors are likely involved.

HOST RANGE, TISSUE TROPISM, RECEPTORS, AND VIRUS ENTRY
FCV is considered to be host specific and to infect only felids. There have been several reports of isolation of FCV-like viruses from dogs with diarrhea, however [42–44]. Sequence analysis of some of these viruses has confirmed their relation to FCV. In none of these cases, however, was it clear that an active calicivirus infection was present. Without conclusive evidence of infection, it remains unclear if FCV can occasionally infect dogs or if the virus can simply pass through the gastrointestinal tract of dogs without initiating infection. Serosurveys in dogs might help to clarify this issue. If dogs can be infected and transmit FCV, this would be important epidemiologically, given the extensive contact between cats and dogs. A survey of human sera from blood donors found that 8.2% (n = 374) of normal human sera and 14% (48 of 350) of sera from clinically normal individuals whose blood was rejected because of high alanine aminotransferase levels had reactivity to FCV antigen [45]; as yet, no human disease is associated with FCV seropositivity. Neutralizing antibodies to FCV have also been found in marine mammals [46]. The fact that serologic evidence of FCV exposure has been found in human beings and marine mammals suggests the range of hosts that FCV can infect may be broader than suspected.

FCV is most commonly associated with vesicular disease. As described previously, however, FCV has also been isolated from cats with a range of different disease syndromes. Many caliciviruses are enteric pathogens; thus, it is interesting that FCV has been isolated from kittens with diarrhea and that some FCV isolates are resistant to bile salt inactivation [47]. In general, FCV is not commonly looked for in fecal samples. It is possible that more virulent isolates of FCV may be passaged through the gastrointestinal tract, however, and may be able to replicate in intestinal epithelial cells in some cases.

The cellular tropism of many viruses is partially determined at the level of virus binding and entry into the host cell [33]. In general, FCV binds poorly to nonfeline cells [48–50]. The block to FCV replication in many nonpermissive cells can be overcome by introducing the viral RNA genome into those cells by transfection [48,51–54]. Thus, the susceptibility of many nonpermissive cells to FCV infection is determined at a stage before delivery of the viral genome into the cytosol. The recent identification of feline junctional adhesion molecule A (JAM-A) and α-2,6 sialic acid as receptors for FCV may help our understanding of its tissue and cellular tropism [49,50]. JAM-A is a member of a family of immunoglobulin-like molecules that are differentially expressed on epithelium, endothelium, platelets, and leukocytes in human beings and mice [55]. The tissue distribution of feline JAM-A has not yet been investigated but would be predicted to be similar. JAM-A localizes to the tight junctional complexes at the intercellular junctions between epithelial and endothelial cells [55]. JAM-A functions to maintain tight junctions and is likely involved in diapedesis of leukocytes [56,57]. Although the presence of α-2,6 sialic acid on the surface of cells enhances FCV binding, it is insufficient to mediate infectious entry [50]. In contrast, expression of feline JAM-A in nonpermissive cell lines confers susceptibility to infection [49].

Two studies have examined the entry pathway of FCV [51,58]. An early study established that FCV infectious entry depends on exposure to low pH, implicating an endosomal uptake pathway [58]. A more recent study using drugs and dominant inhibitors of different endocytic uptake pathways has confirmed that membrane penetration by FCV requires exposure to a low pH environment during cell entry and has shown that FCV is taken into cells by clathrin-mediated uptake from the plasma membrane [51].

Given the variance in tissue targeting among FCV biotypes, one attractive hypothesis is that biotype behavior among FCVs reflects different binding interactions between the virus and a cohort of receptors, such as the JAM family members. In studies on viral distribution of FCV-infected cats, those with oral or lingual ulceration have virus within mucosal and, rarely, respiratory epithelial cells (Patricia A. Pesavento, unpublished data, 2005). In contrast, in cats naturally infected with VS-FCV, viral antigen is present within endothelial and parenchymal cells in addition to epithelial cells [16].

GENOMIC STRUCTURE AND GENETIC VARIABILITY

The genome of FCV is approximately 7.7 kb in length and is an mRNA for open reading frame (ORF) 1 (Fig. 1) [3,59]. ORF1 encodes an approximately 1800 amino-acid polyprotein that is cleaved by a viral proteinase into individual polypeptides that function to form the viral replication complexes [60]. A subgenomic mRNA of approximately 2.4 kb (see Fig. 1) encodes ORF2

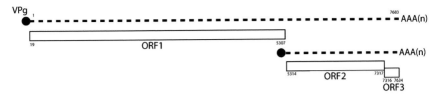

Fig. 1. Genome-translation. Diagram of the FCV genome (Urbana) and ORFs. The dashed lines indicate the genome length and subgenomic RNAs. The filled circle represents the VPg (NS5) protein covalently linked to the 5' end of the genome or subgenome. The three ORFs are indicated below the RNA species from which they are translated. The numbers indicate the first nucleotide of each start (AUG) codon and the beginning and end of the genome.

and ORF3. ORF2 of FCV encodes the precapsid protein (VP1) [61,62], and ORF3 encodes a minor capsid protein (VP2) [63].

The overall identify of FCV genomic nucleotide sequences from isolates collected worldwide is approximately 80%. Despite this high level of diversity, FCV sequences can be categorized into only two distinct genotypes, and only Japanese isolates are present in genotype II [64]. The sequence diversity of FCV occurs because of errors introduced into the genome during viral replication by the viral polymerase and because of recombination between genomes derived from different FCV strains during viral replication [65,66]. A recent longitudinal epidemiologic study in a shelter in the United Kingdom showed that 16 different FCV isolates were cocirculating [67]. The diversity of FCV sequences and the capacity of FCV to undergo rapid evolution explain the emergence of new FCV strains. In addition, this diversity argues strongly for the development of broadly cross-reactive vaccines that can protect not only against disease but against infection.

VIRUS TRANSLATION AND REPLICATION

The calicivirus genome does not have a cap structure or an internal ribosomal entry site. The virus-encoded genome-linked protein (VPg) protein, which is covalently linked at the 5'-end of the virus genome and subgenome, functions to initiate calicivirus RNA translation by recruiting eukaryotic translation initiation factor (eIF) 4E and eIF3 [68–70].

Calicivirus replication occurs in association with intracellular membranes and likely proceeds through a minus strand RNA intermediate that is used as the template for the synthesis of positive-sense full-length genomic and subgenomic RNAs [3]. FCV infection induces apoptosis in Crandell-Reese feline kidney cells (CRFKs) [71]. Like other positive-strand RNA viruses, calicivirus infection leads to inhibition of cellular protein synthesis.

CAPSID STRUCTURE, ANTIGENIC DETERMINANTS, AND ANTIGENIC VARIATION

The FCV capsid serves various functions during the viral life cycle and contains antigenic determinants that are recognized by the host immune system.

Capsid functions include recognition and packaging of the genome, attachment to new susceptible host cells, interaction with specific host cell receptor(s), penetration of the host cell membrane, and delivery of the genome into the cytosol. In addition, the capsid must protect the genome from damage in the environment during transmission from host to host. Experiments to determine the stability of the FCV capsid to various environmental conditions have found that the capsid is relatively stable between a pH of 4 to 8.5 (Ossiboff and John S.L. Parker, unpublished data) [72] and can survive for up to 2 weeks in an infected environment. The FCV capsid is stable in the environment, and practitioners should not be lulled into a false sense of security by the lack of signs of disease in multicat households. A recent study found that 16 different FCV isolates were circulating in a cat shelter that was considered to have "good" biosecurity protocols [67]. The recent outbreaks of virulent systemic FCV and the ease with which the virus was spread by veterinary professionals illustrate the true contagiousness and stability of FCV in general. Human noroviruses are readily spread, and it is estimated that the infectious dose is as little as 10 to 100 virions [3]. Although the infectious dose is not known for FCV, it seems likely that a much lower dose than is normally used in experimental studies can lead to infection and disease. Experiments done by one of the authors and a colleague (R.J. Ossiboff and John S.L. Parker, unpublished data, 2006) have shown that VS-FCV isolates do not differ in their environmental stability from less virulent FCV isolates. Thus, despite the mild clinical signs caused by FCV under most conditions, this virus can be easily spread in the clinic and probably is spread on clothing of veterinarians and technicians. So-called "vaccine-breakdowns" might, in fact, be attributed to infections that were obtained inadvertently at the time of vaccination. A good policy would therefore be to schedule vaccinations for young animals at times when older animals are not present and to ensure that a clean laboratory coat is worn during vaccination clinics. In addition, the use of disposable gloves that are changed between animals seems prudent.

The sequences of FCV capsid-encoding genes (ORF2) show substantial variation. On average, the nucleotide sequence identity of ORF2 is approximately 80%, and the overall amino-acid identity of VP1 is 88% (R.J. Ossiboff and John S.L. Parker, unpublished data, 2006). Although FCV isolates show significant antigenic variation [73–75], serum neutralization studies using various polyclonal antibodies have found substantial cross-reactivity to different isolates [74–76]. Because of this antigenic overlap, all FCV isolates were considered to belong to a single diverse serotype [74]. More recently, Neill and colleagues [78] and Knowles and colleagues [77] have challenged this idea. In a study examining the neutralization patterns of 103 different FCV isolates, Knowles and colleagues [77] found that antisera raised against the F9 vaccine strains crossreacted with 54% of the tested isolates; however, they noted that antisera raised against other field isolates neutralized substantially fewer isolates. Neill and colleagues [78] found markedly altered antigenicity in chimeric viruses, in which the hypervariable regions of the capsid protein were swapped with those of different isolates. Given the diversity of FCV isolates, it seems likely that more than one serotype of FCV exists.

Although it is reasonable to hypothesize that viruses associated with variant diseases might cluster antigenically, numerous attempts to show a correlation between antigenic reactivity and specific FCV-associated diseases or "biotypes" have failed [22,25,79].

The FCV capsid is icosahedral, and its capsomeres have a distinctive cup-like (the name calici- is derived from the Latin word *calyx*, meaning cup-shaped) appearance by negative-stain electron microscopy. The crystallographic structure of the closely related San Miguel Sealion virus 4 (SMSV4) has recently been solved [80], and because of the similarity between the capsid proteins of FCV and SMSV4 ($\sim$52% identity), this structure serves as an important model to predict the structure of the FCV capsid. The capsid is formed from 180 copies of the VP1 capsid protein arranged as 90 arch-like dimers in a T = 3 icosahedral lattice. An analysis of the SMSV4 capsid predicted that the receptor binding site on the capsid would lie at the interface between VP1 dimers. This interface contained conserved residues, whereas the surrounding regions of the dimer had much more variation. The neutralizing epitopes that have been mapped for FCV seem to map to the variable regions of the dimer, which suggests that the antibodies elicited likely select in vivo for capsid variants that can escape neutralization. If this is true, a better vaccine might be developed if an immune response could be elicited against the more conserved regions of the capsid.

References

[1] Oliver SL, et al. Genomic characterization of the unclassified bovine enteric virus Newbury agent-1 (Newbury1) endorses a new genus in the family Caliciviridae. Virology 2006;350(1):240–50.

[2] Faquet CM, editor. Virus taxonomy classification and nomenclature of viruses: the VIIIth report of the International Committee on Taxonomy of Viruses. Oxford:Elsevier/Academic Press; 2005.

[3] Green KY. Caliciviridae: the noroviruses. In: Knipe DM, Howley PM, editors. Field's virology. Philadelphia: Williams & Wilkins; 2007. p. 949–79.

[4] Hurley K, Sykes J. Update on feline calicivirus: new trends. Vet Clin North Am Small Anim Pract 2003;33(4):759–72.

[5] Radford A, et al. Feline calicivirus. Vet Res 2007;38(2):319–35.

[6] Fastier L. New feline virus isolated in tissue culture. Am J Vet Res April 1957;18(67):382–9.

[7] Bannasch MJ, Foley JE. Epidemiologic evaluation of multiple respiratory pathogens in cats in animal shelters. J Feline Med Surg 2005;7(2):109–19.

[8] Cai Y, et al. An etiological investigation of domestic cats with conjunctivitis and upper respiratory tract disease in Japan. J Vet Med Sci 2002;64(3):215–9.

[9] Helps CR, et al. Factors associated with upper respiratory tract disease caused by feline herpesvirus, feline calicivirus, Chlamydophila felis and Bordetella bronchiseptica in cats: experience from 218 European catteries. Vet Rec 2005;156(21):669–73.

[10] Harbour DA, Howard PE, Gaskell RM. Isolation of feline calicivirus and feline herpesvirus from domestic cats 1980 to 1989. Vet Rec 1991;128(4):77–80.

[11] Coyne KP, et al. Long-term analysis of feline calicivirus prevalence and viral shedding patterns in naturally infected colonies of domestic cats. Vet Microbiol 2006;118(1–2):12–25.

[12] Hurley KE, et al. An outbreak of virulent systemic feline calicivirus disease. J Am Vet Med Assoc 2004;224(2):241–9.
[13] Coyne K. Evolutionary mechanisms of persistence and diversification of a calicivirus within endemically infected natural host populations. J Virol 2007;81(4):1961–71.
[14] Coyne K, et al. Lethal outbreak of disease associated with feline calicivirus infection in cats. Vet Rec 2006;158(16):544–50.
[15] Pedersen N, et al. An isolated epizootic of hemorrhagic-like fever in cats caused by a novel and highly virulent strain of feline calicivirus. Vet Microbiol 2000;73(4):281–300.
[16] Pesavento P, et al. Pathologic, immunohistochemical, and electron microscopic findings in naturally occurring virulent systemic feline calicivirus infection in cats. Vet Pathol 2004;41(3):257–63.
[17] Schorr-Evans E, et al. An epizootic of highly virulent feline calicivirus disease in a hospital setting in New England. J Feline Med Surg 2003;5(4):217–26.
[18] Binns SH, et al. A study of feline upper respiratory tract disease with reference to prevalence and risk factors for infection with feline calicivirus and feline herpesvirus. J Feline Med Surg 2000;2(3):123–33.
[19] Dawson S, et al. Acute arthritis of cats associated with feline calicivirus infection. Res Vet Sci 1994;56(2):133–43.
[20] Love DN, Baker KD. Sudden death in kittens associated with a feline picornavirus. Aust Vet J 1972;48(11):643.
[21] Sato Y, et al. Properties of a calicivirus isolated from cats dying in an agitated state. Vet Rec 2004;155(25):800–5.
[22] Dawson S, et al. Typing of feline calicivirus isolates from different clinical groups by virus neutralisation tests. Vet Rec 1993;133(1):13–7.
[23] TerWee J, et al. Comparison of the primary signs induced by experimental exposure to either a pneumotropic or a 'limping' strain of feline calicivirus. Vet Microbiol 1997;56(1–2):33–45.
[24] Knowles JO, et al. Studies on the role of feline calicivirus in chronic stomatitis in cats. Vet Microbiol 1991;27(3–4):205–19.
[25] Poulet H, et al. Comparison between acute oral/respiratory and chronic stomatitis/gingivitis isolates of feline calicivirus: pathogenicity, antigenic profile and cross-neutralisation studies. Arch Virol 2000;145(2):243–61.
[26] Coyne K, et al. Recombination of feline calicivirus within an endemically infected cat colony. J Gen Virol 2006;87(Pt 4):921–6.
[27] Holzinger EA, Kahn DE. Pathologic features of picornavirus infections in cats. Am J Vet Res 1970;31(9):1623–30.
[28] Hoover E, Kahn D. Experimentally induced feline calicivirus infection: clinical signs and lesions. J Am Vet Med Assoc 1975;166(5):463–8.
[29] Langloss J, Hoover E, Kahn D. Ultrastructural morphogenesis of acute viral pneumonia produced by feline calicivirus. Am J Vet Res 1978;39(10):1577–83.
[30] Harrison TM, et al. Systemic calicivirus epidemic in captive exotic felids. J Zoo Wildl Med 2007;38(2):292–9.
[31] Rong S, et al. Characterization of a highly virulent feline calicivirus and attenuation of this virus. Virus Res 2006;122(1–2):95–108.
[32] Ossiboff R, et al. Feline caliciviruses (FCVs) isolated from cats with virulent systemic disease possess in vitro phenotypes distinct from those of other FCV isolates. J Gen Virol 2007;88(Pt 2):506–17.
[33] Nathanson N, Murphy FA. The sequential steps in viral infection. In: Nathanson N, editor. Viral pathogenesis and immunity. 2nd edition. Boston: Elsevier Academic Press; 2007. p. 14–26.
[34] Jazic E, et al. An evaluation of the clinical, cytological, infectious and histopathological features of feline acne. Vet Dermatol 2006;17(2):134–40.

[35] Declercq J. Pustular calicivirus dermatitis on the abdomen of two cats following routine ovariectomy. Vet Dermatol 2005;16(6):395–400.

[36] Sykes JM, et al. Oral eosinophilic granulomas in tigers (Panthera tigris)—a collection of 16 cases. J Zoo Wildl Med 2007;38(2):300–8.

[37] Bennett D, et al. Detection of feline calicivirus antigens in the joints of infected cats. Vet Rec 1989;124(13):329–32.

[38] van Vuuren M, et al. Characterisation of a potentially abortigenic strain of feline calicivirus isolated from a domestic cat. Vet Rec 1999;144(23):636–8.

[39] Tenorio A, et al. Chronic oral infections of cats and their relationship to persistent oral carriage of feline calici-, immunodeficiency, or leukemia viruses. Vet Immunol Immunopathol 1991;29(1–2):1–14.

[40] Lommer MJ, Verstraete FJ. Concurrent oral shedding of feline calicivirus and feline herpesvirus 1 in cats with chronic gingivostomatitis. Oral Microbiol Immunol 2003;18(2):131–4.

[41] Truyen U, Geissler K, Hirschberger J. Tissue distribution of virus replication in cats experimentally infected with distinct feline calicivirus isolates. Berl Munch Tierarztl Wochenschr 1999;112(9):355–8.

[42] Evermann JF, et al. Isolation and identification of caliciviruses from dogs with enteric infections. Am J Vet Res 1985;46(1):218–20.

[43] Gabriel SS, Tohya Y, Mochizuki M. Isolation of a calicivirus antigenically related to feline caliciviruses from feces of a dog with diarrhea. J Vet Med Sci 1996;58(10):1041–3.

[44] Martella V, et al. Analysis of the capsid protein gene of a feline-like calicivirus isolated from a dog. Vet Microbiol 2002;85(4):315–22.

[45] Smith AW, et al. Vesivirus viremia and seroprevalence in humans. J Med Virol 2006;78(5):693–701.

[46] Berke T, et al. Phylogenetic analysis of the caliciviruses. J Med Virol 1997;52(4):419–24.

[47] Mochizuki M. Different stabilities to bile among feline calicivirus strains of respiratory and enteric origin. Vet Microbiol 1992;31(2–3):297–302.

[48] Kreutz LC, Seal BS, Mengeling WL. Early interaction of feline calicivirus with cells in culture. Arch Virol 1994;136(1–2):19–34.

[49] Makino A, et al. Junctional adhesion molecule 1 is a functional receptor for feline calicivirus. J Virol 2006;80(9):4482–90.

[50] Stuart AD, Brown TD. Alpha2,6-linked sialic acid acts as a receptor for feline calicivirus. J Gen Virol 2007;88(Pt 1):177–86.

[51] Stuart AD, Brown TD. Entry of feline calicivirus is dependent on clathrin-mediated endocytosis and acidification in endosomes. J Virol 2006;80(15):7500–9.

[52] Burroughs J, Brown F. Presence of a covalently linked protein on calicivirus RNA. J Gen Virol 1978;41(2):443–6.

[53] Herbert TP, Brierley I, Brown TD. Identification of a protein linked to the genomic and subgenomic mRNAs of feline calicivirus and its role in translation. J Gen Virol 1997;78(Pt 5):1033–40.

[54] Sosnovtsev S, Green K. RNA transcripts derived from a cloned full-length copy of the feline calicivirus genome do not require VPg for infectivity. Virology 1995;210(2):383–90.

[55] Martin-Padura I, et al. Junctional adhesion molecule, a novel member of the immunoglobulin superfamily that distributes at intercellular junctions and modulates monocyte transmigration. J Cell Biol 1998;142(1):117–27.

[56] Petri B, Bixel MG. Molecular events during leukocyte diapedesis. FEBS J 2006;273(19):4399–407.

[57] Nourshargh S, Krombach F, Dejana E. The role of JAM-A and PECAM-1 in modulating leukocyte infiltration in inflamed and ischemic tissues. J Leukoc Biol 2006;80(4):714–8.

[58] Kreutz LC, Seal BS. The pathway of feline calicivirus entry. Virus Res 1995;35(1):63–70.

[59] Carter M, et al. The complete nucleotide sequence of a feline calicivirus. Virology 1992;190(1):443–8.

[60] Sosnovtsev SV, Garfield M, Green KY. Processing map and essential cleavage sites of the nonstructural polyprotein encoded by ORF1 of the feline calicivirus genome. J Virol 2002;76(14):7060–72.

[61] Carter M. Feline calicivirus protein synthesis investigated by Western blotting. Arch Virol 1989;108(1–2):69–79.

[62] Sosnovtsev S, Sosnovtseva S, Green K. Cleavage of the feline calicivirus capsid precursor is mediated by a virus-encoded proteinase. J Virol 1998;72(4):3051–9.

[63] Sosnovtsev SV, et al. Feline calicivirus VP2 is essential for the production of infectious virions. J Virol 2005;79(7):4012–24.

[64] Sato Y, et al. Phylogenetic analysis of field isolates of feline calicivirus (FCV) in Japan by sequencing part of its capsid gene. Vet Res Commun 2002;26(3):205–19.

[65] Jiang X, et al. Characterization of a novel human calicivirus that may be a naturally occurring recombinant. Arch Virol 1999;144(12):2377–87.

[66] Bull R, et al. Norovirus recombination in ORF1/ORF2 overlap. Emerg Infect Dis 2005;11(7):1079–85.

[67] Coyne KP, et al. Longitudinal molecular epidemiological analysis of feline calicivirus infection in an animal shelter: a model for investigating calicivirus transmission within high-density, high-turnover populations. J Clin Microbiol 2007;45(10):3239–44.

[68] Daughenbaugh K, et al. The genome-linked protein VPg of the Norwalk virus binds eIF3, suggesting its role in translation initiation complex recruitment. EMBO J 2003;22(11):2852–9.

[69] Chaudhry Y, et al. Caliciviruses differ in their functional requirements for eIF4F components. J Biol Chem 2006;281(35):25315–25.

[70] Goodfellow I, et al. Calicivirus translation initiation requires an interaction between VPg and eIF 4 E. EMBO Rep 2005;6(10):968–72.

[71] Sosnovtsev S, et al. Feline calicivirus replication induces apoptosis in cultured cells. Virus Res 2003;94(1):1–10.

[72] Lee KM, Gillespie JH. Thermal and pH stability of feline calicivirus. Infect Immun 1973;7(4):678–9.

[73] Kreutz LC, Johnson RP, Seal BS. Phenotypic and genotypic variation of feline calicivirus during persistent infection of cats. Vet Microbiol 1998;59(2–3):229–36.

[74] Povey RC. Serological relationships among feline caliciviruses. Infect Immun 1974;10(6):1307–14.

[75] Kalunda M, et al. Serologic classification of feline caliciviruses by plaque-reduction neutralization and immunodiffusion. Am J Vet Res 1975;36(4 Pt.1):353–6.

[76] Povey C, Ingersoll J. Cross-protection among feline caliciviruses. Infect Immun 1975;11(5):877–85.

[77] Knowles J, et al. Neutralisation patterns among recent British and North American feline calicivirus isolates from different clinical origins. Vet Rec 1990;127(6):125–7.

[78] Neill JD, Sosnovtsev SV, Green KY. Recovery and altered neutralization specificities of chimeric viruses containing capsid protein domain exchanges from antigenically distinct strains of feline calicivirus. J Virol 2000;74(3):1079–84.

[79] Geissler K, et al. Genetic and antigenic heterogeneity among feline calicivirus isolates from distinct disease manifestations. Virus Res 1997;48(2):193–206.

[80] Chen R, et al. X-ray structure of a native calicivirus: structural insights into antigenic diversity and host specificity. Proc Natl Acad Sci U S A 2006;103(21):8048–53.

Vet Clin Small Anim 38 (2008) 787–797

VETERINARY CLINICS
SMALL ANIMAL PRACTICE

Canine Distemper Virus

Vito Martella, DVM, Gabrielle Elia, DVM,
Canio Buonavoglia, DVM*

Department of Animal Health and Wellbeing, Faculty of Veterinary Medicine,
University of Bari, Strada per Casamassima km 3, 70010 Valenzano, Bari, Italy

Canine distemper virus (CDV) belongs to the genus *Morbillivirus*, family Paramyxoviridae, along with phocid distemper virus, measles virus, rinderpest virus, peste-des-petits-ruminants virus, and cetacean Morbilliviruses [1].

CDV is the causative agent of a severe systemic disease in dogs characterized by a variety of symptoms, including fever, respiratory and enteric signs, and neurologic disorders. Clinical disease caused by CDV has been known for centuries and is described unequivocally in books of the seventeenth century, reporting large epidemics all over Europe [2].

The introduction of the modified-live (ML) CDV vaccines in the 1950s and their extensive use has greatly helped to keep the disease under control [3,4]. Notwithstanding, the incidence of CDV-related disease in canine populations throughout the world seems to have increased in the past decades, and several episodes of CDV disease in vaccinated animals have been reported [5,6].

CAUSE

CDV has an enveloped virion containing a nonsegmented negative-stranded RNA genome that encodes for a single-envelope–associated protein (M), two glycoproteins (the hemagglutinin H and the fusion protein F), two transcriptase-associated proteins (the phosphoprotein P and the large protein L), and the nucleocapsid protein (N) that encapsulates the viral RNA [1]. The H gene is a key protein for CDV itself and its animal hosts [3], because the virus uses this protein for attachment to receptors on the cell in the first step of infection. An adequate host immune response against the H protein may prevent CDV infection [7]. After attachment, the F protein promotes fusion of the cell membranes with the viral envelope. The F protein also promotes membrane fusion between the host cells, with formation of syncytia [8].

Field CDV strains do not replicate well in vitro, and virus adaptation to tissue cell cultures is fastidious. Canine or ferret macrophages may be used for adaptation of CDV to grow in vitro, whereas for propagation of cell-adapted CDV

*Corresponding author. E-mail address: c.buonavoglia@veterinaria.uniba.it (C. Buonavoglia).

0195-5616/08/$ – see front matter
doi:10.1016/j.cvsm.2008.02.007

strains (used in the vaccines), canine kidney cell lines or Vero cells are used. Because the signaling lymphocyte activation molecule (SLAM) acts as a receptor for CDV, Vero cells expressing canine SLAM (VeroDog SLAM tag) have been engineered that allow efficient isolation of field CDV strains [9]. CDV replication in cells usually induces formation of giant cells (syncytia) with intracytoplasmatic and intranuclear eosinophilic inclusion bodies (Figs. 1 and 2).

EPIDEMIOLOGY

CDV has a broad host range, and evidence for the infection has been obtained in several mammalian species in the families Canidae, Mustelidae, Procyonidae, Ursidae, and Viverridae. The infection has also been described in captive and free-ranging large felids [10–12], in captive Japanese primates [13], in collared peccaries [14], and in Siberian seals [15].

Like other enveloped viruses, CDV is quickly inactivated in the environment and transmission mainly occurs by direct animal-to-animal contact or by exposure to infectious aerosol. The virus can be detected at high titers from secretions and excretions, including urine [16]. Routine disinfections and cleaning readily abolish virus infectivity.

Temporal fluctuations in disease prevalence have been observed, with increased frequency during the cold season. Age-related susceptibility to infection (3–6-month-old pups are more susceptible than older dogs) correlates with the decline in maternally derived immunity, because young pups are protected by passive immunity and most adult dogs are protected by vaccine immunization.

CDV is a monotypic virus, as defined by polyclonal antisera, although a variety of biotypes exist that differ in their pathogenic patterns [17]. Molecular techniques are useful to study virus epidemiology and to investigate the dynamics of circulation of the various strains in susceptible animals. Comparative studies of CDV strains have revealed that the H gene is subjected to higher genetic and antigenic variation than other CDV genes. The amino acid sequence

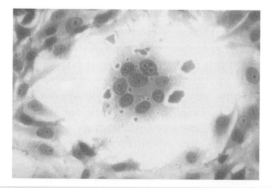

Fig. 1. Vero cells infected by CDV. There is formation of giant cells (syncytia) with intracytoplasmatic and intranuclear eosinophilic inclusion bodies.

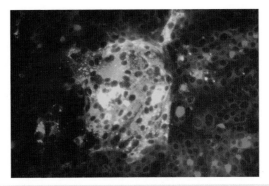

Fig. 2. Vero cells infected by CDV. The focus of viral replication is revealed by immunofluorescence.

of the F protein shows approximately 4% variability among different CDV strains, which is in the range of variability of the other structural proteins, whereas the CDV H proteins vary by approximately 10%. Sequence variation in the H protein may affect neutralization-related sites with disruption of important epitopes. Based on the pronounced genetic diversity in the H gene, it is possible to characterize most CDV field strains into six major genetic lineages, referred to as America-1 and -2, Asia-1 and -2, European, and Arctic [18–22], that are variously distributed according to geographic patterns but irrespective of the species of origin. The greatest genetic and antigenic diversity is between the vaccine strains (America-1 lineage) and the other CDV lineages [5,23–27]. Sera raised against field CDV isolates may have neutralizing titers up to 10-fold higher against the homologous virus than against vaccine strains [10]. Although it is unlikely that such antigenic variations may affect the protection induced by vaccine immunization, it is possible that critical amino acid substitutions in key epitopes of the H protein may allow escape from the limited antibody repertoire of maternal origin of young unvaccinated pups, increasing the risk for infection by field CDV strains. Some CDV strains seem to be more virulent or are associated with different tropism, but this relies on individual variations among the various strains rather than on peculiar properties inherent to a given CDV lineage [17,28].

CLINICAL SIGNS AND PATHOLOGIC FINDINGS

The virus enters the new host by the nasal or oral route and promptly starts replication in the lymphoid tissues [29], resulting in severe immunosuppression. T cells are more affected than B cells [30]. The decrease in CD4+ lymphocytes is quick and persists for several weeks. Because the percentage of CDV-infected lymphocytes is low, the mechanisms of immunosuppression are not clear. Immunosuppressive activity has been displayed by the N protein of measles virus, and the same mechanisms likely trigger immunosuppression in CDV infection [31,32].

The incubation period may range from 1 to 4 weeks or more. Transient fever reaches a peak 3 to 6 days after infection and is associated with the initial virus spread in the body. Loss of appetite, slight depression, ocular and nasal discharge, and tonsillitis may be observed (Fig. 3). By days 6 to 9 after infection, CDV spreads by cell-associated viremia to the epithelial cells in most organs [33,34].

At this stage, the outcome of the infection and the severity of the signs vary markedly on the basis of strain virulence, the age of the animal, and the immune status. If the dog develops a strong immune response, the virus gets cleared from the tissues and the animal completely recovers from the infection. When dogs develop a weak immune response, the virus is able to reach the epithelial tissues and the central nervous system (CNS). The initial clinical signs disappear, but the virus persists for extended periods in the uvea, neurons, or urothelium and in some skin areas (foot pads). The CNS signs are delayed, and hyperkeratosis is observed in some dogs. In the dogs that fail to mount an immune response, the virus continues to replicate and spreads massively throughout the body. Localization in the CNS results in acute demyelinization, and most dogs die 2 to 4 weeks after the infection [34,35].

As a result of the epithelial localization, respiratory, intestinal, and dermatologic signs occur by 10 days after infection. The symptoms are often exacerbated by secondary bacterial infections and include purulent nasal discharge, coughing, dyspnea, pneumonia, diarrhea, vomiting, and dermal pustules. Enamel hypoplasia and hyperkeratosis of the foot pads and nose are typical signs of CDV infection and may be observed in dogs that survive subclinical or subacute infections (Figs. 4 and 5) [36].

Starting from 20 days after infection, neurologic signs may be observed, such as circling, head tilt, nystagmus, partial or complete paralysis, convulsions, and

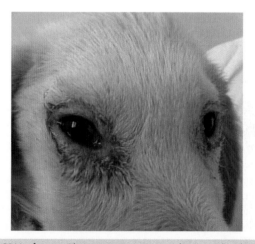

Fig. 3. Dog with CDV infection. There is conjunctivitis with periocular discharge.

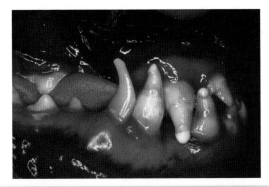

Fig. 4. Dog with CDV infection. There is marked enamel hypoplasia.

dementia. Involuntary jerky twitching or contraction of muscles and convulsions preceded by chewing-gum movements of the mouth are considered typical of CDV infection. Neurologic signs may also be observed at 40 to 50 days after infection as a consequence of chronic CDV-induced demyelination. The virus persists in the CNS, and the disease evolves discontinuously but progressively. Some dogs may still recover, but compulsive movements (eg, head pressing, continual pacing, uncoordinated hypermetria) tend to persist [36].

Intracytoplasmic eosinophilic inclusion bodies are present in the epithelial cells of the skin, bronchi, intestinal tract, urinary tract, bile duct, salivary glands, adrenal glands, CNS, lymph nodes, and spleen [36].

Demyelination is the prominent lesion in the brain of dogs that are infected with CDV. In acute infection, primary demyelination is not related to inflammation [37], because perivascular cuffs are not visible, and it is likely accounted for by metabolic dysfunction with decreased myelin synthesis in CDV-infected oligodendrocytes and by virus-induced activation of microglial cells [38].

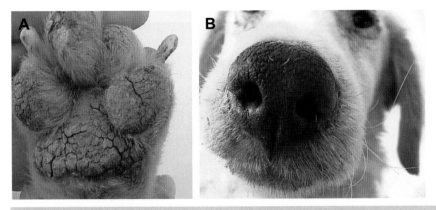

Fig. 5. Dog with CDV infection. There is hyperkeratosis of the foot pads (A) and nose (B).

In chronic forms of disease, the demyelination lesions are attributable to an inflammatory reaction elicited by a CDV-specific immune response and by persistence of CDV infection in the tissues. Experiments in vitro suggest that chronic inflammatory demyelination is attributable to an "innocent bystander mechanism" resulting from interactions between macrophages and virus-antibody complexes [39]. Perivascular cuffing with lymphocytes, plasma cells, and monocytes is present in the areas of demyelination.

A rare outcome of CDV infection is chronic encephalomyelitis of mature dogs, termed *old dog encephalitis* (ODE) [40]. ODE presents as a progressive cortical derangement with a wide range of clinical signs and usually occurs in dogs with a complete vaccination history. Frequent lesions associated with ODE are multifocal perivascular and parenchymal lymphoplasmacytic encephalitis in the cerebral hemispheres. The disease seems to develop in dogs after acute CDV infection when the virus gains the capability to persist in the nervous tissues. An ODE-like disease has been reproduced experimentally in a gnotobiotic dog infected with a neurovirulent CDV strain [41]. The molecular mechanisms triggering persistence of CDV in the CNS are not clear. Changes in proteins H, F, and M, or in their interactions, may affect CDV fusogenicity in vitro and are likely involved in the genesis of ODE [42,43].

DIAGNOSIS

CDV should be considered in the diagnosis of any febrile condition of puppies with multisystemic symptoms. Several laboratory tests are available to confirm CDV infection. Immunofluorescence (IF) on conjunctival, nasal, and vaginal smears (Fig. 6) is not sensitive and can detect CDV antigens only within 3 weeks after infection, when the virus is still present in the epithelial cells [3]. Virus isolation on cell lines from clinical or autoptic samples (eg, conjunctival swabs, buffy coat, spleen and lung tissues) is fastidious. Molecular assays, such as reverse transcriptase polymerase chain reaction (RT-PCR) [44–47] and real-time RT-PCR [16], are sensitive and specific. A nested RT-PCR system

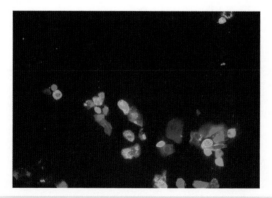

Fig. 6. IF examination for CDV on a conjunctival smear from a dog.

with specific probes allows characterization of the various CDV lineages and distinction between field and vaccine CDV strains [48].

High antibody titers to CDV may be detected for several months after vaccination or after subclinical or clinical infection by ELISA, virus neutralization, or indirect IF assays. Virus-specific immunoglobulin M (IgM) persists for at least 3 months after infection and may be specifically recognized by ELISA [49,50] and used as a marker of recent CDV infection.

TREATMENT AND PREVENTION

Treatment consists of supportive care and antibiotics and is aimed at preventing the secondary bacterial infections that are frequent in immunosuppressed animals. Ribavirin, a purine nucleoside analogue, is capable of inhibiting CDV replication in vitro [51], but antiviral drugs are not available commercially.

ML vaccines are recommended for immunization of dogs. The vaccines elicit long-lasting protective immunity. Several vaccine strains (eg, Onderstepoort, Rockborn, Snyder Hill) have been used [3]. Some CDV vaccine strains may retain pathogenicity when used in wild-life animals [52] or when administered in conjunction with canine adenovirus-type 1 [53,54]. Also, immune depression induced by stress or by concomitant diseases may result in reversion to virulence of the vaccine [55,56]. Although vaccine-induced disease is always suspected in dogs that develop distemper shortly after immunization, in most cases, the disease is induced by wild-type CDV infecting pups before active immunization is elicited. Vaccine failures are mostly attributable to incorrect vaccinal protocols or to vaccine alteration after improper storage.

A recombinant viral vaccine for CDV has also been produced [57]. The vaccine proved to be effective and safe, because the virus vector does not replicate efficiently in mammals.

A major problem encountered in CDV vaccination of young pups is the lingering passive immunity of maternal origin that may prevent active immunization. Because measles virus is closely related to CDV, heterologous vaccination with the human Morbillivirus has been adopted to immunize pups in the face of maternally derived immunity. The vaccine seems to have limited efficacy [58] and introduces a human pathogen into the environment. The vaccine is not authorized in Europe, although it is available in the United States.

To overcome the interference of maternally derived antibodies, pups should be vaccinated with ML CDV vaccine at 6 to 8 weeks of age and again after 2 to 4 weeks. Annual revaccination is usually performed. Because protective immunity induced by ML vaccines persists for more than 3 years [59], vaccination of the animals is recommended every 3 years.

SUMMARY

Vaccine-based prophylaxis has greatly helped to keep distemper disease under control [3,4]. Notwithstanding, the incidence of CDV-related disease in canine populations throughout the world seems to have increased in the past decades, and several episodes of CDV disease in vaccinated animals have been reported [5,6], with nation-wide proportions in some cases [60]. In parallel, in the past decades, uncontrolled trading of low-cost and high-value breed pets from countries with low sanitation standards has been intensifying in several European countries, leading to emergence or re-emergence of infectious threats to the health of dogs [61]. Recently, the spread of unusual CDV strains (termed *Arctic* after their similarity to CDV strains identified in animals of the Arctic ecosystem) has been documented in Europe, and similar CDV strains have been identified in North America [22,62,63]. The reasons for and effects of these changes in CDV epidemiology are unknown. Increasing surveillance should be pivotal to identify new CDV variants and to understand the dynamics of CDV epidemiology. In addition, it is important to evaluate whether the efficacy of the vaccine against these new strains may somehow be affected.

References

[1] van Regenmortel HVM, Fauquet CM, Bishop DHL, et al, editors. Virus taxonomy. Seventh report of the International Committee on Taxonomy of Viruses. New York: Academic Press; 2000. p. 556–7.

[2] Blancou J. Dog distemper: imported into Europe from South America? Hist Med Vet 2004;29:35–41.

[3] Appel MJ. Canine distemper virus. In: Appel MJ, editor. Virus infection of carnivores. Amsterdam: Elsevier; 1987. p. 133–59.

[4] Appel MJ, Summers BA. Pathogenicity of Morbilliviruses for terrestrial carnivores. Vet Microbiol 1995;44:187–91.

[5] Blixenkrone-Møller M, Svansson V, Appel M, et al. Antigenic relationship between field isolates of Morbilliviruses from different carnivores. Arch Virol 1992;123:279–94.

[6] Decaro N, Camero M, Greco G, et al. Canine distemper and related diseases: report of a severe outbreak in a kennel. New Microbiol 2004;27:177–81.

[7] von Messling V, Zimmer G, Herrler G, et al. The hemagglutinin of canine distemper virus determines tropism and cytopathogenicity. J Virol 2001;75(14):6418–27.

[8] Lamb RA, Paterson RG, Jardetzky TS. Paramyxovirus membrane fusion: lessons from the F and HN atomic structures. Virology 2006;344:30–7.

[9] Seki F, Ono N, Yamaguchi R, et al. Efficient isolation of wild strains of canine distemper virus in Vero cells expressing canine SLAM (CD150) and their adaptability to marmoset B95a cells. J Virol 2003;77:9943–50.

[10] Harder TC, Kenter M, Vos H, et al. Canine distemper virus from diseased large felids: biological properties and phylogenetic relationships. J Gen Virol 1996;77:397–405.

[11] Roelke-Parker ME, Munson L, Packer C, et al. A canine distemper virus epidemic in Serengeti lions (*Panthera leo*). Nature 1996;379(6564):441–5.

[12] Van de Bildt MW, Kuiken T, Visee AM, et al. Distemper outbreak and its effect on African wild dog conservation. Emerg Infect Dis 2002;8:211–3.

[13] Yoshikawa Y, Ochikubo F, Matsubara Y, et al. Natural infection with canine distemper virus in a Japanese monkey (*Macaca fuscata*). Vet Microbiol 1989;20(3):193–205.

[14] Appel MJ, Reggiardo C, Summers BA, et al. Canine distemper virus infection and encephalitis in javelinas (collared peccaries). Arch Virol 1991;119(1–2):147–52.

[15] Likhoshway YeV, Grachev MA, Kumarev VP, et al. Baikal seal virus. Nature 1989;339(6222):266.

[16] Elia G, Decaro N, Martella V, et al. Detection of canine distemper virus in dogs by real-time RT-PCR. J Virol Methods 2006;136:171–6.

[17] Summers BA, Greisen HA, Appel MJ. Canine distemper encephalomyelitis: variation with virus strain. J Comp Pathol 1984;94:65–75.

[18] Bolt G, Jensen TD, Gottschalck E, et al. Genetic diversity of the attachment (H) protein gene of current field isolates of canine distemper virus. Gen Virol 1997;78:367–72.

[19] Carpenter MA, Appel MJ, Roelke-Parker ME, et al. Genetic characterization of canine distemper virus in Serengeti carnivores. Vet Immunol Immunopathol 1998;65:259–66.

[20] Haas L, Martens W, Greiser-Wilke I, et al. Analysis of the haemagglutinin gene of current wild-type canine distemper virus isolates from Germany. Virus Res 1997;48:165–71.

[21] Harder TC, Kenter M, Vos H, et al. Immunohistochemical analysis of the lymphoid organs of dogs naturally infected with canine distemper virus. J Comp Pathol 1995;113:185–90.

[22] Martella V, Cirone F, Elia G, et al. Heterogeneity within the hemagglutinin genes of canine distemper virus (CDV) strains detected in Italy. Vet Microbiol 2006;116(4):301–9.

[23] Harder TC, Klusmeyer K, Frey H-R, et al. Intertypic differentiation and detection of intratypic variants among canine and phocid distemper Morbillivirus isolates by kinetic neutralization using a novel immunoplaque assay. J. Virol. Methods 1993;41:77–92.

[24] Iwatsuki K, Tokiyoshi S, Hirayama N, et al. Antigenic difference in the H proteins of canine distemper viruses. Vet Microbiol 2000;71:281–6.

[25] Örvell C, Blixenkrone-Møller M, Svansson V, et al. Immunological relationships between phocid and canine distemper virus studied with monoclonal antibodies. J Gen Virol 1990;71:2085–92.

[26] Gemma T, Iwatsuki K, Shin YS, et al. Serological analysis of canine distemper virus using an immunocapture ELISA. J Vet Med Sci 1996;58:791–4.

[27] Mochizuki M, Motoyoshi M, Maeda K, et al. Complement-mediated neutralization of canine distemper virus in vitro: cross-reaction between vaccine Onderstepoort and field KDK-1 strains with different hemagglutinin gene characteristics. Clin Diagn Lab Immunol 2002;9:921–4.

[28] Lednicky JA, Dubach J, Kinsel MJ, et al. Genetically distant American canine distemper virus lineages have recently caused epizootics with somewhat different characteristics in raccoons living around a large suburban zoo in the USA. Virol J 2004;1:2.

[29] Appel MJ. Pathogenesis of canine distemper. Am J Vet Res 1969;30:1167–82.

[30] Iwatsuki K, Okita M, Ochikubo F, et al. Immunohistochemical analysis of the lymphoid organs of dogs naturally infected with canine distemper virus. J Comp Pathol 1995;113(2):185–90.

[31] Marie JC, Saltel F, Escola JM, et al. Cell surface delivery of the measles virus nucleoprotein: a viral strategy to induce immunosuppression. J Virol 2004;78(21):11952–61.

[32] Kerdiles YM, Cherif B, Marie JC, et al. Immunomodulatory properties of Morbillivirus nucleoproteins. Viral Immunol 2006;19(2):324–34.

[33] Appel MJ, Shek WR, Summers BA. Lymphocyte-mediated immune cytotoxicity in dogs infected with virulent canine distemper virus. Infect Immun 1982;37(2):592–600.

[34] Winters KA, Mathes LE, Krakowka S, et al. Immunoglobulin class response to canine distemper virus in gnotobiotic dogs. Vet Immunol Immunopathol 1984;5(2):209–15.

[35] Appel MJ, Mendelson SG, Hall WW. Macrophage Fc receptors control infectivity and neutralization of canine distemper virus-antibody complexes. J Virol 1984;51(3):643–9.

[36] Green EC, Appel MJ. Canine distemper virus. In: Green, editor. Infections diseases of the dog and cat. Philadelphia: W.B. Saunders company; 1990. p. 226–41.

[37] Vandevelde M, Kristensen F, Kristensen B, et al. Immunological and pathological findings in demyelinating encephalitis associated with canine distemper virus infection. Acta Neuropathol 1982;56:1–8.

[38] Vandevelde M, Zurbriggen A. Demyelination in canine distemper virus infection: a review. Acta Neuropathol (Berl) 2005;109:56–68.

[39] Griot C, Burge T, Vandevelde M, et al. Antibody-induced generation of reactive oxygen radicals by brain macrophages in canine distemper encephalitis: a mechanism for bystander demyelination. Acta Neuropathol (Berl) 1989;78:396–403.

[40] Lincoln SD, Gorham JR, Davis WC, et al. Etiological studies of old dog encephalitis. I. Demosntration of canine distemper viral antigen in the brain of two cases. Vet Pathol 1971; 8:1–8.

[41] Axthelm MK, Krakowka S. Experimental old dog encephalitis (ODE) in a gnotobiotic dog. Vet Pathol 1998;35:527–34.

[42] Plattet P, Rivals JP, Zuber B, et al. The fusion protein of wild-type canine distemper virus is a major determinant of persistent infection. Virology 2005;337:312–26.

[43] Plattet P, Cherpillod P, Wiener D, et al. Signal peptide and helical bundle domains of virulent canine distemper virus fusion protein restrict fusogenicity. J Virol 2007;81:11413–25.

[44] Frisk AL, Konig M, Moritz A, et al. Detection of canine distemper virus nucleoprotein RNA by reverse transcription-PCR using serum, whole blood, and cerebrospinal fluid from dogs with distemper. J Clin Microbiol 1999;37(11):3634–43.

[45] Rzeżutka A, Mizak B. Application of N-PCR for diagnosis of distemper in dogs and fur animals. Vet Microbiol 2002;88:95–103.

[46] Saito TB, Alfieri AA, Wosiacki SR, et al. Detection of canine distemper virus by reverse transcriptase-polymerase chain reaction in the urine of dogs with clinical signs of distemper encephalitis. Res Vet Sci 2006;80:116–9.

[47] Shin YJ, Cho KO, Cho HS, et al. Comparison of one-step RT-PCR and a nested PCR for the detection of canine distemper virus in clinical samples. Aust Vet J 2004;82:83–6.

[48] Martella V, Elia G, Lucente MS, et al. Genotyping canine distemper virus (CDV) by a heminested multiplex PCR provides a rapid approach for investigation of CDV outbreaks. Vet Microbiol 2007;122:32–42.

[49] Blixenkrone-Møller M, Pedersen IR, Appel MJ, et al. Detection of IgM antibodies against canine distemper virus in dog and mink sera employing enzyme-linked immunosorbent assay (ELISA). J Vet Diagn Invest 1991;3:3–9.

[50] von Messling V, Harder TC, Moennig V, et al. Rapid and sensitive detection of immunoglobulin M (IgM) and IgG antibodies against canine distemper virus by a new recombinant nucleocapsid protein-based enzyme-linked immunosorbent assay. J Clin Microbiol 1999;37: 1049–56.

[51] Elia G, Belloli C, Cirone F, et al. In vitro efficacy of ribavirin against canine distemper virus. Antiviral Res 2008;77(2):108–13.

[52] Durchfeld B, Baumgärtner W, Herbst W, et al. Vaccine-associated canine distemper infection in a litter of African hunting dogs (Lycaon pictus). Zentralbl Veterinarmed B 1990;37(3):203–12.

[53] Cornwell HJ, Thompson H, McCandlish IA, et al. Encephalitis in dogs associated with a batch of canine distemper (Rockborn) vaccine. Vet Rec 1988;122(3):54–9.

[54] McCandlish IA, Cornwell HJ, Thompson H, et al. Distemper encephalitis in pups after vaccination of the dam. Vet Rec 1992;130(2):27–30.

[55] Max JG, Appel MJ. Reversion to virulence of attenuated canine distemper virus in vivo and in vitro. J Gen Virol 1978;41:385–93.

[56] Krakowka S, Olsen RG, Axthelm M, et al. Canine parvovirus infection potentiates canine distemper encephalitis attributable to modified live-virus vaccine. J Am Vet Med Assoc 1982;180(2):137–9.

[57] Pardo MC, Bauman JE, Mackowiak M. Protection of dogs against canine distemper by vaccination with a canarypox virus recombinant expressing canine distemper virus fusion and hemagglutinin glycoproteins. Am J Vet Res 1997;58:833–6.

[58] Appel MJ, Shek WR, Shesberadaran H, et al. Measles virus and inactivated canine distemper virus induce incomplete immunity to canine distemper. Arch Virol 1984;82(1–2): 73–82.

[59] Gore TC, Lakshmanan N, Duncan KL, et al. Three-year duration of immunity in dogs following vaccination against canine adenovirus type-1, canine parvovirus, and canine distemper virus. Vet Ther 2005;6:5–14.
[60] Ek-Kommonen C, Sihvonen L, Pekkanen K, et al. Outbreak of canine distemper in vaccinated dogs in Finland. Vet Rec 1997;141:380–3.
[61] Decaro N, Campolo M, Elia G, et al. Infectious canine hepatitis: an "old" disease reemerging in Italy. Res Vet Sci 2007;83:269–73.
[62] Pardo ID, Johnson GC, Kleiboeker SB. Phylogenetic characterization of canine distemper viruses detected in naturally infected dogs in North America. J Clin Microbiol 2005;43(10):5009–17.
[63] Demeter Z, Lakatos B, Palade EA, et al. Genetic diversity of Hungarian canine distemper virus strains. Vet Microbiol 2007;122:258–69.

Vet Clin Small Anim 38 (2008) 799–814

VETERINARY CLINICS
SMALL ANIMAL PRACTICE

Canine Adenoviruses and Herpesvirus

Nicola Decaro, DVM, Vito Martella, DVM,
Canio Buonavoglia, DVM*

Department of Animal Health and Wellbeing, Faculty of Veterinary Medicine, University of Bari,
Strada per Casamassima km 3, 70010 Valenzano, Bari, Italy

C anine adenoviruses (CAVs) and canine herpesvirus (CHV) are pathogens of dogs that have been known for several decades. The two distinct types of CAVs, type 1 (CAV-1) and type 2 (CAV-2), are
responsible for infectious canine hepatitis (ICH) and infectious tracheobronchitis (ITB), respectively [1,2]. Systematic vaccination of dogs has considerably reduced circulation of CAVs in canine populations, although severe outbreaks
can be still observed in countries in which CAV vaccines are not used routinely
or as a consequence of uncontrolled importation of dogs from endemic areas.
CHV can be detected in healthy dogs or in association with different clinical
forms, chiefly with mortality in newborns and with respiratory disease or genital lesions in adult dogs [3]. CHV vaccination is not applied routinely, and the
infection is common in kenneled dogs.

In the present article, the currently available literature on CAVs and CHV is
reviewed, providing a meaningful update on the epidemiologic, pathogenetic,
clinical, diagnostic, and prophylactic aspects of the infections caused by these
important pathogens.

CANINE ADENOVIRUSES
Cause and History
ICH, formerly known as epizootic encephalitis of foxes [1], was first observed
in dogs in 1930 [2]. The causative agent CAV-1 was isolated a decade later [4]
and was attenuated through passages on canine and swine cell lines to produce
vaccines [5,6]. CAV-2 was first recovered in 1961 from dogs with laryngotracheitis [7]. The isolate, strain Toronto A26/61, was initially considered to be
an attenuated strain of CAV-1; only subsequently was it proposed as the prototype of a distinct CAV designated as CAV-2 [8–12].

CAV-1 and CAV-2 are members of the genus *Mastadenovirus*, family Adenoviridae, and are closely related antigenically [13,14] and genetically (75% identity at
the nucleotide level) [15,16]. Despite their antigenic and genetic relatedness, they
are easily distinguishable by restriction endonuclease analysis [17,18] and DNA

*Corresponding author. E-mail address: c.buonavoglia@veterinaria.uniba.it (C. Buonavoglia).

0195-5616/08/$ – see front matter
doi:10.1016/j.cvsm.2008.02.006

hybridization [19]. They also exhibit different hemagglutination patterns and cell tropism. CAV-1 recognizes the vascular endothelial cells and hepatic and renal parenchymal cells as targets for viral replication, whereas CAV-2 replicates efficiently in the respiratory tract and, to a limited extent, in the intestinal epithelia [20–22].

Infection by CAVs has been described worldwide in several mammalian species. Dogs, red foxes, wolves, and coyotes are highly susceptible to CAV infection [3]. The overall prevalence of antibodies to CAVs in European red foxes (*Vulpes vulpes*) in Australia was 23.2%, with marked geographic, seasonal, and age differences [23], whereas the prevalence of antibody was 97% in island foxes (*Urocyon littoralis*) in the Channel Islands, California [24]. Antibodies to CAVs were also detected in free-ranging terrestrial carnivores and marine mammals in Alaska and Canada, including black bears (*Ursus americanus*), fishers (*Martes pennanti*), polar bears (*Ursus maritimus*), wolves (*Canis lupus*), walruses (*Odobenus rosmarus*), and Steller sea lions (*Eumetopias jubatus*) [25,26]. Recently, a fatal CAV-1 infection has been reported in a Eurasian river otter (*Lutra lutra*) [27].

Canine Infectious Hepatitis: Clinical Signs and Pathologic Findings

Canine ICH is a systemic disease described in Canidae and Ursidae. CAV-1 replication in vascular endothelial cells and hepatocytes produces acute necro-hemorrhagic hepatitis, and the disease is more severe in young animals [28,29]. Transmission occurs through animal-to-animal contact or indirectly through exposure to infectious saliva, feces, urine, or respiratory secretions. CAV-1 is shed in urine up to 6 to 9 months after infection [30]. The incubation period in dogs is 4 to 6 days after ingestion of infectious material and 6 to 9 days after direct contact with infected dogs [31]. The mortality rate is 10% to 30% [32]. Coinfections with canine coronavirus (CCoV) [33,34], canine distemper virus (CDV) [34–37], or canine parvovirus [34] can exacerbate the disease, increasing the mortality rates.

Fever (>40°C) is the earliest clinical sign and displays a biphasic course. After the first febrile peak (1–2 days), some dogs recover from the infection. Dogs displaying a second peak of hyperthermia frequently undergo a more severe form of ICH. Commonly observed symptoms are depression, loss of appetite, increased heart rate, hyperventilation, vomiting, and diarrhea. Abdominal pain and distention can occur as a result of accumulation of serosanguineous or hemorrhagic fluid and enlargement of the liver. Frequently, hemorrhagic diathesis is observed with epistaxis, congestion, or hemorrhage of the mucous membranes and skin. Respiratory distress can also be observed as a consequence of laryngitis, tracheitis, and, less frequently, pneumonia. Neurologic signs (hypersalivation, ataxia, and seizures) are rare in dogs and are associated with vascular damage in the central nervous system (CNS) [28,38]. Corneal opacity ("blue eye"; Fig. 1) and interstitial nephritis may occur 1 to 3 weeks after recovery because of deposition of immune complexes [39–41]. Hematologic findings include leukopenia (<2000 cells/μL of blood; mainly attributable to

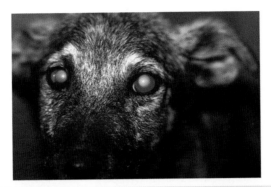

Fig. 1. Dog with ICH. Note bilateral corneal opacity.

a decrease in neutrophil count), increase in the serum transaminases (only in the severe forms of disease) [42], and coagulation disorders associated with disseminated intravascular coagulation (DIC; thrombocytopenia, altered platelet formation, and prolonged prothrombin time) [43]. Proteinuria (albuminuria) can easily reach values greater than 50 mg/dL because of immunomediated glomerulonephritis [29].

At necropsy, the dogs that die during the acute phase of the disease often appear in good nutritional state. External examination can reveal ecchymoses and petechial hemorrhages, whereas the abdominal cavity contains abundant clear or serosanguineous fluid. The liver is enlarged, yellowish brown, congested, and spotted with small rounding areas of necrosis; the gallbladder appears thickened, edematous, and grayish or bluish white opaque in color (Fig. 2). Edema of the gallbladder wall is a constant finding. Congestion and hemorrhagic lesions are observed in the spleen, lymph nodes (Fig. 3), thymus, pancreas, and kidneys. Lungs show patchy areas of consolidation

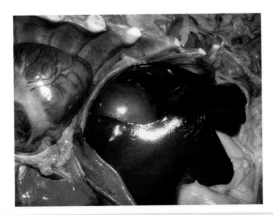

Fig. 2. Dog with ICH. There is marked enlargement of the gallbladder.

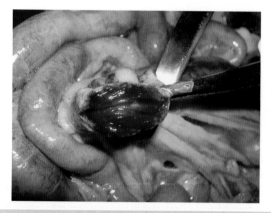

Fig. 3. Dog with ICH. The lymph node is enlarged and hemorrhagic.

because of bronchopneumonia. Hemorrhagic enteritis can also be observed (Fig. 4) [3,28].

Histologic changes in the liver are characterized by centrolobular necrosis, along with neutrophilic and mononuclear cell infiltration and intranuclear inclusions in the Kupffer's cells and hepatocytes. Multifocal areas of congestion, hemorrhage, and leukocyte infiltration can be observed in several organs, mainly in the liver and kidneys, because of vascular damage and inflammation. Interstitial nephritis and iridocyclitis with corneal edema are also present in dogs recovering from ICH [44].

Infectious Tracheobronchitis: Clinical Signs and Pathologic Findings

The route of infection by CAV-2 is oronasal. Respiratory signs are consistent with damage of bronchial epithelial cells. CAV-2 infections rarely result in

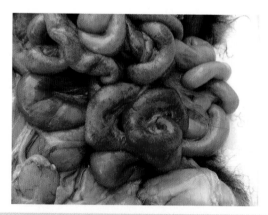

Fig. 4. Dog with ICH. There is segmental hemorrhagic enteritis.

overt clinical signs, however, despite the presence of extensive lung lesions. Clinical signs typical of ITB are observed when CAV-2 infection is complicated by other viral or bacterial pathogens of dogs, including canine parainfluenza 3 virus [45], CDV [46–48], *Bordetella bronchiseptica* [49], mycoplasmas [50,51], and *Streptococcus equi* subsp. *zooepidemicus* [52–54]. In addition, other viruses with tropism for the respiratory tract have been recently identified and associated with ITB-like forms in dogs, such as influenza A virus [54,55], a pantropic variant of CCoV [56], and the canine respiratory coronavirus (CRCoV) [57,58]. CHV and mammalian reoviruses have rarely been reported from dogs with ITB and likely do not play a major role in the disease complex [59,60].

ITB (kennel cough) is an acute and highly contagious respiratory disease of dogs affecting the larynx, trachea, bronchi, and, occasionally, lower respiratory tract [61]. Kennel cough is typically a complex of diseases caused by viral pathogens (eg, CAVs, CHV, canine parainfluenza virus, reoviruses) in association with bacteria, mainly *B bronchiseptica* and *Mycoplasma* spp. Most frequently, a dry hacking cough is observed as a consequence of an uncomplicated, self-limiting, and primarily viral infection of the trachea and bronchi. In complicated forms, which are more common in pups and immunocompromised dogs, secondary bacterial infections and involvement of pulmonary tissue overlap the viral infection. Cough is usually associated with mucoid discharges. The condition may progress to bronchopneumonia and, in the most severe instances, death [61]. Usually, CNS involvement is not seen, although death in pups with neurologic disease associated with CAV-2 infection has been reported [62].

At postmortem examination, red areas of consolidation can be observed in the lungs, especially in the complicated forms. Histologically, necrotizing bronchitis and bronchiolitis obliterans may be observed. Infection of type 2 alveolar cells is associated with interstitial pneumonia and the presence of viral inclusion bodies in their nuclei [63–68].

Diagnosis, Treatment, and Vaccination

Hematologic findings (eg, leukopenia, prolonged blood clotting, increased activities of alanine aminotransferase [ALT] and aspartate aminotransferase [AST]) may be indicative of CAV-1 infection, although the increase of transaminases is commonly observed only in severely affected or moribund dogs. Postmortem findings and histopathologic changes are highly suggestive of CAV-1 infection. Confirmation of a diagnosis of ICH is obtained by virus isolation on permissive cell lines, such as Madin Darby canine kidney (MDCK) cells. A polymerase chain reaction (PCR) protocol has recently been developed for molecular diagnosis [69]. Ocular swabs, feces, and urine can be collected in vivo for virus isolation and PCR. Postmortem samples can be withdrawn from the kidney, lung, and lymphoid tissues. The liver is rich in arginase, which inhibits viral growth in cell cultures [70], but it represents the most important organ for histopathologic examination [28,29]. Viral growth in cells is revealed by rounding cells that form clusters and detach from the monolayers [34]. Immunofluorescence (IF) can detect viral antigens in infected cell cultures and in acetone-fixed tissue sections or smears. Viral replication can also be demonstrated by detection of nuclear inclusion bodies in the cells after hematoxylin-eosin staining.

Neither virus isolation nor IF is able to distinguish between the two adenovirus types. Because CAV-2 can also be detected in the internal organs and feces of vaccinated or acutely infected dogs [46] and CAV-1 is also frequently isolated from respiratory secretions, trachea, and lungs, distinction between CAV-1 and CAV-2 necessarily deserves laboratory examination. Restriction fragment length polymorphism analysis on viral genomes using the endonucleases *Pst*I and *Hpa*II generates differential patterns [17,18]. Detection and differentiation of CAV-1 and CAV-2 by PCR with a single primer pair are also possible [69]. Although CAVs agglutinate erythrocytes of several species, hemagglutination is not used in routine diagnosis [71]. Because most dogs are vaccinated and CAV-2 infection is frequent in dogs, serology has low diagnostic relevance [21,39].

Treatment of ICH is primarily symptomatic and supportive. Dehydration and DIC require administration of fluids, plasma, or whole-blood transfusions and anticoagulants. Hyperammonemia attributable to hepatic and renal damages can be corrected by oral administration of nonabsorbable antibiotics and lactulose and by oral or parenteral administration of potassium and urinary acidificants (ascorbic acid). Supportive therapy may facilitate the clinical recovery of infected dogs, provided that there is time for hepatocellular regeneration [29].

Uncomplicated forms of CAV-2–associated ITB can be treated with glucocorticoids, antitussives, and bronchodilators as cough suppressants. Aerosol therapy can be effective in dogs displaying excessive accumulation of tracheal and bronchial secretions. Antimicrobial therapy is recommended in the complicated forms and when the lower respiratory tract seems to be involved [29].

Use of vaccines has greatly reduced the burden of ICH in canine populations. Initial attempts were made with CAV-1 inactivated vaccines, which require repeated inoculations [72]. CAV-1–based modified-live virus (MLV) vaccines proved to be highly effective but were associated with interstitial nephritis and corneal opacity [22]. Administration of CAV-1 in conjunction with CDV vaccines was also associated with postvaccinal encephalitis [73]. Because CAV-1 and CAV-2 are able to confer cross-protection, the current vaccines contain MLV CAV-2, which is not able to induce renal or ocular damage. The CAV-2 attenuated strain Toronto A26/61 is contained in most vaccine formulations [22,74]. In the absence of maternally derived antibodies (MDAs), a single dose administered subcutaneously or intramuscularly is protective against ICH and ITB. Because of the possible interference of MDAs, however, the vaccination schedule requires administration of at least two vaccine doses at a 3- to 4-week interval, starting when pups are 8 to 10 weeks old. Intranasal administration of an MLV CAV-2 vaccine has been proposed to overcome MDA interference, but it may be associated with the onset of mild respiratory disease [29].

Vaccination is usually repeated yearly, although after administration of two doses of CAV-2 vaccine, immunity seems to persist for more than 3 years [75,76]. Although extensive vaccination has greatly reduced the incidence of CAV infections, re-emergence of ICH has been described in Italy, likely as the result of parallel trading of pups with uncertain sanitary status from Eastern European countries [34]. At the moment, there are few data on the molecular epidemiology of CAVs, but it is commonly accepted that vaccine breaks occur rarely with CAV vaccines, because the viruses are genetically stable. Accordingly, CAV infection in vaccinated dogs has been associated with MDA interference in the early life of the pups rather than with emergence of variants genetically distant from the prototype strains contained in CAV-2 vaccines [34].

CANINE HERPESVIRUS
Cause
CHV was first described in the mid-1960s as the causative agent of a fatal septicemic disease of puppies [77]. CHV is included in the Alphaherpesvirinae subfamily, Herpesviridae family [78]. The virus is sensitive to lipid solvents, is readily inactivated at temperatures greater than 40°C, and is rapidly inactivated by common disinfectants.

CHV seems to be a monotypic virus, as defined by antigenic comparison of various isolates [77,79]. The genome structure of CHV resembles that of other members of the Alphaherpesvirus subfamily [80–83]. Southern blot hybridization and sequence analysis of various genes have shown a close genetic relatedness to feline herpesvirus (FHV-1), to phocid herpesvirus 1, and to the equid herpesviruses 1 and 4 [84–86].

Epidemiology
The host range of CHV is restricted to dogs [87]. Antibodies to CHV have been detected in sera of European red foxes (*V vulpes*) in Australia [23] and Germany [88], however, and in sera of North American river otters (*Lontra canadensis*) from New York [89], whereas a CHV-like virus has been isolated from captive coyote pups [90].

The virus seems to be present worldwide in domestic and wild dogs. Serologic surveys have shown a relatively high prevalence of CHV in household and colony-bred dogs. The prevalence of antibodies in dogs was 88% in England, 45.8% in Belgium, and 39.3% in The Netherlands [91–93]. Serologic studies in Italy have revealed a high prevalence in kenneled dogs (27.9%), whereas the prevalence was lower in pets (3.1%) [94]. In the United States, Fulton and colleagues [95] studied the prevalence of antibodies against CHV in Washington and found only a 6% seroprevalence. Transmission occurs by direct contact with oronasal or genital secretions, because CHV is quickly inactivated in the environment.

Clinical Signs and Pathogenesis
The age of the pups at the time of infection is critical for the outcome of the disease. Infection of susceptible puppies at 1 to 2 weeks of age may be associated

with fatal generalized necrotizing and hemorrhagic disease, whereas infection of pups older than 2 weeks of age and adult dogs is often asymptomatic [77]. Infection in older dogs seems to be restricted to the upper respiratory tract [96]. Also, CHV has been identified in corneal swabs of adult dogs with corneal ulcerations [97]. Transplacental transmission of CHV and fetal death may also occur [98], and CHV infection is suspected in dogs with fertility disorders. The high susceptibility of newborn pups to fatal acute CHV-induced disease is likely related to the fact that pups have low and poorly regulated body temperature and CHV growth is optimal at lower than normal body temperature [99].

Neonatal mortality
CHV infection is generally fatal in neonatal pups lacking maternally derived immunity. Death of 1- to 4-week-old pups is most common. Neonatal pups may be infected during passage through the birth canal or by contact with oronasal secretions of other dogs. The duration of illness in newborn pups is 1 to 3 days. Signs include vocalization, anorexia, dyspnea, abdominal pain, incoordination, and soft feces, whereas the rectal temperature is not elevated and may be low. Serous or hemorrhagic nasal discharge and petechial hemorrhage on the mucous membranes may also be observed.

In pups less than 1 week of age at the time of infection, CHV replicates in the nasal mucosa, pharynx, and tonsils before spreading by means of the blood (in macrophages) to the liver, kidneys, lymphatic tissues, lungs, and CNS. The incubation period is approximately 6 to 10 days. Death in affected litters usually occurs over a period of a few days to a week. Litter mortality can reach a peak of 100%. In pups older than 2 to 3 weeks of age at the time of infection, CHV infection is generally asymptomatic, although CNS signs, including blindness and deafness, have been described [100].

Reproductive disorders
CHV can cause occasional in utero infections that result in death of the fetus or pup shortly after birth [77,98]. Pregnant dogs infected at midgestation or later may abort weak or stillborn pups. Pups may seem normal at parturition but die within a few days of birth. The infected dams develop protective immunity, and CHV-related diseases are not observed in subsequent litters because maternally derived immunity protects the pups during the first week of life when they are most susceptible.

Primary genital infections in susceptible adult animals may be associated with lymphofollicular lesions and vaginal hyperemia (Fig. 5). Male animals may have similar lesions over the base of the penis and the prepuce.

Respiratory disease
CHV has been detected in dogs with ITB [101], but its role remains controversial. Experimental infection has been shown to cause mild clinical symptoms of rhinitis and pharyngitis [96] or tracheobronchitis [102]. Experimental infection by the intravenous route in adult foxes resulted in fever, lethargy, and respiratory signs, although peroral infection did not [103].

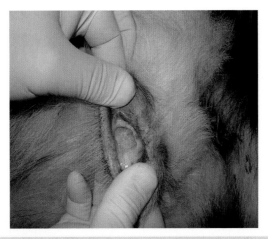

Fig. 5. Dog with primary genital herpesvirus infection. There is lymphoid hyperplasia and hyperemia of the vaginal mucosa.

A long-term survey in a population of dogs in a shelter has demonstrated CHV in 9.6% of lung and 12.8% of tracheal samples. CHV infections occurred later than other viral infections. CHV was detected more frequently at weeks 3 and 4 after a dog's introduction in the kennel, whereas CRCoV and canine parainfluenza were detected more frequently within the first and second weeks, respectively. Interestingly, CHV infection was apparently related to more severe respiratory signs [53]. In a 1-year study in training centers for working dogs, however, seroconversion to CHV seemed to be more frequent in dogs infected with CRCoV [104], suggesting virus reactivation after disease-induced stress.

Latency

After symptomatic and asymptomatic infections, dogs remain latently infected and virus may be excreted at unpredictable intervals over periods of several months or years. Reactivation of latent virus may be provoked by environmental or social stress or, experimentally, by immunosuppressive drugs (corticosteroids) or antilymphocyte serum. Latent virus persists in the trigeminal ganglia and other sites, such as lumbosacral ganglia, tonsils, and parotid salivary glands [3,105–107]. Latently infected dogs represent a source of infection for susceptible animals, and this is of particular concern in breeding dogs that can ensure CHV transmission through genital secretions.

Pathologic Findings

Multifocal areas of necrosis and hemorrhage may be observed in most organs, including the lungs, liver, brain, and intestine, with the kidneys being the most classic organ affected. Circumscribed areas of hemorrhage and necrosis on a pale gray cortex give the organs a spotted appearance (Fig. 6). Lymph nodes and spleens appear enlarged. Meningoencephalitis also is common. Necrosis in

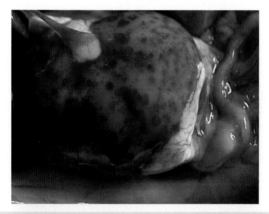

Fig. 6. Puppy with neonatal herpesvirus infection. There is multifocal hemorrhage and necrosis of the kidneys.

the placenta is observed in infected pregnant animals. Fetal lesions are similar to those seen in affected puppies.

Diagnosis, Treatment, and Vaccination

Diagnosis of CHV infection may be achieved by isolation of the virus on permissive cell lines. The virus can be adapted for growth on canine primary or secondary kidney or testicular cells and in canine cell lines. Growth is optimal at 34°C to 35°C, with diminished virus yields at temperatures higher than 36°C. In cell cultures, virus growth is revealed by formation of typical clusters of rounded cells that tend to detach, and for certain isolates, by formation of syncytia with type A intranuclear inclusions. PCR assays are available, significantly increasing diagnostic reliability and sensitivity [107]. Serologic screenings to evaluate the neutralizing antibodies may be useful to investigate the presence of CHV in kennels.

Because CHV growth is optimal at temperatures lower than 36°C [99], attempts were made to influence the evolution of CHV-induced disease in experimentally infected pups. Experimentally infected newborn pups reared at elevated temperatures that raised their body temperature to 38.5°C to 39.5°C survived CHV infection but presented with permanent neurologic damage [108]. Likewise, residual neurologic damage may be observed in infected dogs treated with antiviral drugs, such as vidarabine. Accordingly, neither artificial temperature nor vidarabine may be applied for the therapy of CHV.

An inactivated subunit vaccine is available commercially in Europe. The vaccine should be administered to bitches during heat or the initial stages of pregnancy and again at the sixth to seventh week of gestation. A temperature-resistant mutant of CHV attenuated through serial cell passages has been proposed as an MLV vaccine [109], but its safety and efficacy have not been evaluated and such a vaccine is not available commercially.

SUMMARY

CAV infections have been satisfactorily controlled in the past decades as a consequence of the vaccination programs adopted in all developed countries. Nevertheless, there are some concerns about the possible introduction of infected dogs from areas of uncertain epidemiologic conditions, in which both CAV types are widespread as a result of the lack of systematic canine immunization [34]. CAV vaccines have been proved to be safe and effective for prevention of ICH and ITB, conferring protection against more recent CAV strains, albeit prepared with old CAV-2 strains [28,110].

Conversely, CHV is still circulating in canine populations worldwide, mainly in shelters and breeding kennels. Active immunization is recommended in pregnant bitches to prevent fatal infections in newborn pups [111]. When the MDAs decrease, however, pups born to vaccinated bitches become susceptible and, along with unvaccinated dogs, maintain CHV infection. It is unclear whether vaccination prevents CHV infection and virus shedding through secretions. In addition, control of the infection is hindered by the fact that CHV is often associated with asymptomatic infections, and the real prevalence of CHV infection is likely underestimated [87].

The intensification of surveillance activity using new diagnostic techniques and molecular analysis tools may help to investigate the epidemiology of CAV and CHV infections more thoroughly and to plan adequate measures of control.

References

[1] Green RG, Ziegler NR, Breen BB, et al. Epizootic fox encephalitis. I. General description. Am J Hyg 1930;12:109–29.
[2] Cowdry EV, Scott GH. A comparison of certain intranuclear inclusions found in the livers of dogs without history of infection with intranuclear inclusions characteristic of the action of filtrable viruses. Arch Pathol 1930;9:1184–96.
[3] Carmichael LE, Greene CE. Canine herpesvirus infection. In: Greene CE, editor. Infectious diseases of the dog and cat. Philadelphia: WB Saunders Co; 1998. p. 28–32.
[4] Cabasso VJ, Stebbins MR, Nortor TW, et al. Propagation of infectious canine hepatitis virus in tissue culture. Proc Soc Exp Biol Med 1954;85:239–45.
[5] Fieldsteel AH, Emery JB. Cultivation and modification of infectious canine hepatitis virus in roller tube cultures of dog kidney. Proc Soc Exp Biol Med 1954;86:819–23.
[6] Cabasso VJ, Stebbins MR, Avampato JM. A bivalent live virus vaccine against canine distemper (CD) and infectious canine hepatitis (ICH). Proc Soc Exp Biol Med 1958;99:46–51.
[7] Ditchfield J, MacPherson LW, Zbitnew A. Association of a canine adenovirus (Toronto A26/61) with an outbreak of laryngotracheitis (kennel cough). A preliminary report. Can Vet J 1962;3:238–47.
[8] Yamamoto R, Marusyk RG. Morphological studies of a canine adenovirus. J Gen Virol 1968;2:191–4.
[9] Fairchild GA, Cohen D. Serologic study of a canine adenovirus (Toronto A26/61) infection in dog. Am J Vet Res 1969;30:923–8.
[10] Swango LJ, Eddy GA, Binn LN. Serologic comparisons of infectious canine hepatitis and Toronto A26/61 canine adenoviruses. Am J Vet Res 1969;30:1381–7.
[11] Marusyk RG, Norrby E, Lundqvist U. Biophysical comparison of two canine adenoviruses. J Virol 1970;5:507–12.

[12] Marusyk RG. Comparison of the immunological properties of two canine adenoviruses. Can J Microbiol 1972;18:817–23.

[13] Matthews REF. Classification and nomenclature of viruses. Intervirology 1982;17:4–199.

[14] Wigand R, Bartha A, Dreizin RS, et al. Adenoviridae: second report. Intervirology 1982;18:169–76.

[15] Morrison MD, Onions DE, Nicolson L. Complete DNA sequence of canine adenovirus type 1. J Gen Virol 1997;78:873–8.

[16] Davison AJ, Benko M, Harrach B. Genetic content and evolution of adenoviruses. J Gen Virol 2003;84:2895–908.

[17] Assaf R, Marsolais G, Yelle J, et al. Unambiguous typing of canine adenovirus isolates by deoxyribonucleic acid restriction-endonuclease analysis. Can J Comp Med 1983;47:460–3.

[18] Hamelin C, Marsolais G, Assaf R. Interspecific differences between DNA restriction profiles of canine adenovirus. Experientia 1984;40:482.

[19] Marusyk RG, Hammarskjold ML. The genetic relationship of two canine adenoviruses as determined by nucleic acid hybridization. Microbios 1972;5:259–64.

[20] Swango LJ, Wooding WL, Binn LN. A comparison of the pathogenesis and antigenicity of infectious canine hepatitis virus and the A26/61 virus strain (Toronto). J Am Vet Med Assoc 1970;156:1687–96.

[21] Marusyk RG, Yamamoto T. Characterization of canine adenovirus hemagglutinin. Can J Microbiol 1971;17:151–5.

[22] Appel M, Bistner SI, Menegus M, et al. Pathogenicity of low-virulence strains of two canine adenoviruses. Am J Vet Res 1973;34:543–50.

[23] Robinson AJ, Crerar SK, Waight Sharma N, et al. Prevalence of serum antibodies to canine adenovirus and canine herpesvirus in the European red fox (Vulpes vulpes) in Australia. Aust Vet J 2005;83:356–61.

[24] Garcelon DK, Wayne RK, Gonzales BJ. A serologic survey of the island fox (Urocyon littoralis) on the Channel Islands, California. J Wildl Dis 1992;28:223–9.

[25] Burek KA, Gulland FM, Sheffield G, et al. Infectious disease and the decline of Steller sea lions (Eumetopias jubatus) in Alaska, USA: insights from serologic data. J Wildl Dis 2005;41:512–24.

[26] Philippa JDW, Leighton PJ, Nielsen O, et al. Antibodies to selected pathogens in free-ranging terrestrial carnivores and marine mammals in Canada. Vet Rec 2004;155:135–40.

[27] Park NY, Lee MC, Kurkure NV, et al. Canine adenovirus type 1 infection of a Eurasian river otter (Lutra lutra). Vet Pathol 2007;44:536–9.

[28] Appel M. Canine adenovirus type 1 (infectious canine hepatitis virus). In: Appel M, editor. Virus infections of carnivores. Amsterdam: Elsevier Science Publishers; 1987. p. 29–43.

[29] Greene CE. Infectious canine hepatitis. In: Greene CE, editor. Infectious diseases of the dog and cat. Philadelphia: WB Saunders; 1990. p. 242–51.

[30] Poppensiek GC, Baker JA. Persistence of virus in urine as factor in spread of infectious hepatitis in dogs. Proc Soc Exp Biol Med 1951;77:279–81.

[31] Baker JA, Richards MG, Brown AL, et al. Infectious hepatitis in dogs. In: Proc Am Vet Med Assoc 87th Ann. Mtg. 1950. p. 242–8.

[32] Cabasso VJ. Infectious canine hepatitis virus. Ann N Y Acad Sci 1962;101:498–514.

[33] Pratelli A, Martella V, Elia G, et al. Severe enteric disease in an animal shelter associated with dual infection by canine adenovirus type 1 and canine coronavirus. J Vet Med B Infect Dis Vet Public Health 2001;48:385–92.

[34] Decaro N, Campolo M, Elia G, et al. Infectious canine hepatitis: an "old" disease reemerging in Italy. Res Vet Sci 2007;83:269–73.

[35] Stookey JL, VanZwieten MJ, Witney GD. Dual viral infections in two dogs. J Am Vet Med Assoc 1972;61:1117–21.

[36] Ducatelle R, Maenhout D, Coussement W, et al. Dual adenovirus and distemper virus pneumonia in a dog. Vet Q 1982;4:84–8.

[37] Kobayashi Y, Ochiai K, Itakura C. Dual infection with canine distemper virus and infectious canine hepatitis virus (canine adenovirus type 1) in a dog. J Vet Med Sci 1993;55: 699–701.

[38] Caudell D, Confer AW, Fulton RW, et al. Diagnosis of infectious canine hepatitis virus (CAV-1) infection in puppies with encephalopathy. J Vet Diagn Invest 2005;17:58–61.

[39] Carmichael LE. The pathogenesis of ocular lesions of infectious canine hepatitis. I. Pathology and virological observation. Pathol Vet 1964;1:73–95.

[40] Carmichael LE. The pathogenesis of ocular lesions of infectious canine hepatitis. II. Experimental ocular hypersensitivity produced by the virus. Pathol Vet 1965;2:344–59.

[41] Wright NG. Canine adenovirus: its role in renal and ocular disease: a review. J Small Anim Pract 1976;17:25–33.

[42] Beckett SD, Burns MJ, Clark CH. A study of the blood glucose, serum transaminase, and electrophoretic patterns of dogs with infectious canine hepatitis. Am J Vet Res 1964;25: 1186–90.

[43] Wigton DH, Kociba GJ, Hoover EA. Infectious canine hepatitis: animal model for viral-induced disseminated intravascular coagulation. Blood 1976;47:287–96.

[44] Carmichael LE, Medic BLS, Bistner SI, et al. Viral-antibody complexes in canine adenovirus type 1 (CAV 1) ocular lesion: leukocyte chemotaxis and enzyme release. Cornell Vet 1975;65:331–51.

[45] Binn LN, Eddy GA, Lazar EC, et al. Viruses recovered from laboratory dogs with respiratory disease. Proc Soc Exp Biol Med 1967;126:140–5.

[46] Decaro N, Camero M, Greco G, et al. Canine distemper and related diseases: report of a severe outbreak in a kennel. New Microbiol 2004;27:177–81.

[47] Chvala S, Benetka V, Mostl K, et al. Simultaneous canine distemper virus, canine adenovirus type 2, and Mycoplasma cynos infection in a dog with pneumonia. Vet Pathol 2007;44:508–12.

[48] Rodriguez-Tovar LE, Ramirez-Romero R, Valdez-Nava Y, et al. Combined distemper-adenoviral pneumonia in a dog. Can Vet J 2007;48:632–4.

[49] Bemis DA, Carmichael LE, Appel M. Naturally occurring respiratory disease in a kennel caused by Bordetella bronchiseptica. Cornell Vet 1977;67:282–93.

[50] Randolph JF, Moise NS, Scarlett JM, et al. Prevalence of mycoplasmal and ureaplasmal recovery from tracheobronchial lavages and of mycoplasmal recovery from pharyngeal swab specimens in cats with or without pulmonary disease. Am J Vet Res 1993;54: 897–900.

[51] Chalker VJ, Owen WM, Paterson C, et al. Mycoplasmas associated with canine infectious respiratory disease. Microbiology 2004;150:3491–7.

[52] Chalker VJ, Brooks HW, Brownlie J. The association of Streptococcus equi subsp. zooepidemicus with canine infectious respiratory disease. Vet Microbiol 2003;95:149–56.

[53] Erles K, Dubovi EJ, Brooks HW, et al. Longitudinal study of viruses associated with canine infectious respiratory disease. J Clin Microbiol 2004;42:4524–9.

[54] Yoon K-J, Cooper VL, Schwartz KJ, et al. Influenza virus infection in racing greyhounds. Emerg Infect Dis 2005;11:1974–5.

[55] Crawford PC, Dubovi EJ, Castleman WL, et al. Transmission of equine influenza virus to dogs. Science 2005;310:482–5.

[56] Buonavoglia C, Decaro N, Martella V, et al. Canine coronavirus highly pathogenic for dogs. Emerg Infect Dis 2006;12:492–4.

[57] Erles K, Toomey C, Brooks HW, et al. Detection of a group 2 coronavirus in dogs with canine infectious respiratory disease. Virology 2003;310:216–23.

[58] Decaro N, Desario C, Elia G, et al. Serological and molecular evidence that canine respiratory coronavirus is circulating in Italy. Vet Microbiol 2007;121:225–30.

[59] Karpas A, King NW, Garcia FG, et al. Canine tracheobronchitis; isolation and characterization of the agent with experimental reproduction of the disease. Proc Soc Exp Biol Med 1968;127:45–52.

[60] Lou TY, Wenner HA. Natural and experimental infection of dogs with reovirus type 1: pathogenicity of the strain for other animals. Am J Hyg 1963;77:293–304.

[61] Appel M, Binn LN. Canine infectious tracheobronchitis. Short review: kennel cough. In: Appel M, editor. Virus infections of carnivores. Amsterdam: Elsevier Science Publisher; 1987. p. 201–11.

[62] Benetka V, Weissenbock H, Kudielka I, et al. Canine adenovirus type 2 infection in four puppies with neurological signs. Vet Rec 2006;158:91–4.

[63] Appel M, Picherill RH, Menegus M, et al. Current status of canine respiratory disease. In: Proc. 20th Gaines Vet Symp. Manhattan: 1970. p. 15–23.

[64] Curtis R, Jemmet JE, Furminger IGS. The pathogenicity of an attenuated strain of canine adenovirus type 2 (CAV-2). Vet Rec 1978;103:380–1.

[65] Appel M. Canine infectious tracheobronchitis (kennel cough): a status report. Compendium on Continuing Education 1981;3:70–9.

[66] Appel M. Canine adenovirus type 2 (infectious laryngotracheitis virus). In: Appel M, editor. Virus infections of carnivores. Amsterdam: Elsevier Science Publisher; 1987. p. 45–51.

[67] Koptopoulos G, Cornwell HJC. Canine adenoviruses: a review. Vet Bull 1981;51: 135–42.

[68] Castleman WL. Bronchiolitis obliterans and pneumonia induced in young dogs by experimental adenovirus infection. Am J Pathol 1985;119:495–504.

[69] Hu RL, Huang G, Qiu W, et al. Detection and differentiation of CAV-1 and CAV-2 by polymerase chain reaction. Vet Res Commun 2001;25:77–84.

[70] Carmichael LE. Identification of a canine adenovirus (infectious canine hepatitis virus) inhibitor in dog liver extracts as arginase. Infect Immun 1972;6:348–54.

[71] Fastier LB. Studies on the hemagglutinin of infectious canine hepatitis virus. J Immunol 1957;78:413–8.

[72] Miller ASH, Curtis R, Furminger IGS. Persistence of immunity to infectious canine hepatitis using a killed vaccine. Vet Rec 1980;106:343–4.

[73] Cornwell HJ, Thompson H, McCandlish IA, et al. Encephalitis in dogs associated with a batch of canine distemper (Rockborn) vaccine. Vet Rec 1998;122:54–9.

[74] Appel M, Carmichael LE, Robson DS. Canine adenovirus type 2-induced immunity to two canine adenoviruses in pups with maternal antibody. Am J Vet Res 1975;36:1199–202.

[75] Gill M, Srinivas J, Morozov I, et al. Three-year duration of immunity for canine distemper, adenovirus, and parvovirus after vaccination with a multivalent canine vaccine. International Journal of Applied Research in Veterinary Medicine 2004;2:227–34.

[76] Gore TC, Coyne MJ, Duncan KL, et al. Three-year duration of immunity in dogs following vaccination against canine adenovirus type-1, canine parvovirus, and canine distemper virus. Vet Ther 2005;6:5–14.

[77] Carmichael LE, Squire RA, Krook L. Clinical and pathologic features of a fatal viral disease of newborn pups. Am J Vet Res 1965;26:803–14.

[78] Virus taxonomy. Seventh report of the International Committee on Taxonomy of Viruses. In: van Regenmortel MHV, Fauquet CM, Bishop DHL, et al, editors. New York: Academic Press; 2000.

[79] Poste G, Lecatsas G, Apostolov K. Electron microscope study of the morphogenesis of a new canine herpesvirus in dog kidney cells. Arch Gesamte Virusforsch 1972;39:317–29.

[80] Rémond M, Sheldrick P, Lebreton F, et al. Gene organization in the UL region and inverted repeats of the canine herpesvirus genome. J Gen Virol 1996;77:37–48.

[81] Haanes EJ, Tomlinson CC. Genomic organization of the canine herpesvirus US region. Virus Res 1998;53:151–62.

[82] Limbach KJ, Limbach MP, Conte D, et al. Nucleotide sequence of the genes encoding the canine herpesvirus gB, gC and gD homologues. J Gen Virol 1994;75:2029–39.

[83] Reubel GH, Pekin J, Webb-Wagg K, et al. Nucleotide sequence of glycoprotein genes B, C, D, G, H and I, the thymidine kinase and protein kinase genes and gene homologue UL24 of an Australian isolate of canine herpesvirus. Virus Genes 2002;25:195–200.

[84] Rota PA, Maes RK. Homology between feline herpesvirus-1 and canine herpesvirus. Arch Virol 1990;115:139–45.

[85] Willoughby K, Bennett M, McCracken CM, et al. Molecular phylogenetic analysis of felid herpesvirus 1. Vet Microbiol 1999;69:93–7.

[86] Martina BE, Harder TC, Osterhaus AD. Genetic characterization of the unique short segment of phocid herpesvirus type 1 reveals close relationships among alpha herpesviruses of hosts of the order Carnivora. J Gen Virol 2003;84:1427–30.

[87] Appel MJ. Canine herpesvirus. In: Appel MJ, editor. Virus infections of carnivores. Amsterdam: Elsevier; 1987. p. 5–15.

[88] Truyen U, Muller T, Heidrich R, et al. Survey on viral pathogens in wild red foxes (Vulpes vulpes) in Germany with emphasis on parvoviruses and analysis of a DNA sequence from a red fox parvovirus. Epidemiol Infect 1998;121:433–40.

[89] Kimber KR, Kollias GV, Dubovi EJ. Serologic survey of selected viral agents in recently captured wild North American river otters (Lontra canadensis). J Zoo Wildl Med 2000;31:168–75.

[90] Evermann JF, LeaMaster BR, McElwain TF, et al. Natural infection of captive coyote pups with a herpesvirus antigenically related to canine herpesvirus. J Am Vet Med Assoc 1984;185:1288–90.

[91] Reading MJ, Field HJ. Detection of high levels of canine herpes virus-1 neutralising antibody in kennel dogs using a novel serum neutralisation test. Res Vet Sci 1999;66:273–5.

[92] Ronsse V, Verstegen J, Onclin K, et al. Seroprevalence of canine herpesvirus-1 in the Belgian dog population in 2000. Reprod Domest Anim 2002;37:299–304.

[93] Rijsewijk FA, Luiten EJ, Daus FJ, et al. Prevalence of antibodies against canine herpesvirus 1 in dogs in The Netherlands in 1997–1998. Vet Microbiol 1999;65:1–7.

[94] Sagazio P, Cirone F, Pratelli A, et al. Infezione da herpesvirus del cane: diffusione sierologica in Puglia. Obiettivi e Documenti Veterinari 1998;5:63–7.

[95] Fulton RW, Ott WL, Duenwald JC, et al. Serum antibodies against canine respiratory viruses: prevalence among dogs of eastern Washington. Am J Vet Res 1974;35:853–5.

[96] Appel MJ, Menegus M, Parsonson IM, et al. Pathogenesis of canine herpesvirus in specific-pathogen-free dogs: 5- to 12-week-old pups. Am J Vet Res 1969;30:2067–73.

[97] Ledbetter EC, Riis RC, Kern TJ, et al. Corneal ulceration associated with naturally occurring canine herpesvirus-1 infection in two adult dogs. J Am Vet Med Assoc 2006;229:376–84.

[98] Hashimoto A, Hirai K, Yamaguchi T, et al. Experimental transplacental infection of pregnant dogs with canine herpesvirus. Am J Vet Res 1982;43:844–50.

[99] Lust G, Carmichael LE. Suppressed synthesis of viral DNA, protein and mature virions during replication of canine herpesvirus at elevated temperature. J Infect Dis 1971;124:572–80.

[100] Carmichael LE. Herpesvirus canis: aspects of pathogenesis and immune response. J Am Vet Med Assoc 1970;156:1714–21.

[101] Binn LN, Alford JP, Marchwicki RH, et al. Studies of respiratory disease in random-source laboratory dogs: viral infections in unconditioned dogs. Lab Anim Sci 1979;29:48–52.

[102] Karpas A, Garcia FG, Calvo F, et al. Experimental production of canine tracheobronchitis (kennel cough) with canine herpesvirus isolated from naturally infected dogs. Am J Vet Res 1968;29:1251–7.

[103] Reubel GH, Pekin J, Venables D, et al. Experimental infection of European red foxes (Vulpes vulpes) with canine herpesvirus. Vet Microbiol 2001;83:217–33.

[104] Erles K, Brownlie J. Investigation into the causes of canine infectious respiratory disease: antibody responses to canine respiratory coronavirus and canine herpesvirus in two kennelled dog populations. Arch Virol 2005;150:1493–504.

[105] Miyoshi M, Ishii Y, Takiguchi M, et al. Detection of canine herpesvirus DNA in the ganglionic neurons and the lymph node lymphocytes of latently infected dogs. J Vet Med Sci 1999;61:375–9.

[106] Okuda Y, Ishida K, Hashimoto A, et al. Virus reactivation in bitches with a medical history of herpesvirus infection. Am J Vet Res 1993;54:551–4.

[107] Burr PD, Campbell ME, Nicolson L, et al. Detection of canine herpesvirus 1 in a wide range of tissues using the polymerase chain reaction. Vet Microbiol 1996;53:227–37.

[108] Carmichael LE, Barnes FD, Percy DH. Temperature as a factor of resistance of young puppies to canine herpesvirus. J Infect Dis 1969;120:669–78.

[109] Carmichael LE, Medic BLS. Small-plaque variant of canine of canine herpesvirus with reduced pathogenicity for newborn pups. Infect Immun 1978;20:108–14.

[110] Day MJ, Horzinek MC, Schultz RD. Guidelines for the vaccination of dogs and cats. Compiled by the vaccination guidelines group (VGG) of the world small animal veterinary association (WSAVA). J Small Anim Pract 2007;48:528–41.

[111] Poulet H, Guigal PM, Soulier M, et al. Protection of puppies against canine herpesvirus by vaccination of the dams. Vet Rec 2001;148:691–5.

Vet Clin Small Anim 38 (2008) 815–825

VETERINARY CLINICS
SMALL ANIMAL PRACTICE

Canine Respiratory Coronavirus: An Emerging Pathogen in the Canine Infectious Respiratory Disease Complex

Kerstin Erles, DrMedVet*,
Joe Brownlie, BVSc, PhD, DSc, FRCPath, FRCVS

Department of Pathology and Infectious Diseases, The Royal Veterinary College, Hawkshead Lane, Hatfield, AL9 7TA, UK

Respiratory disease in dogs is generally of greatest importance in establishments in which dogs are housed in groups, such as shelters, boarding kennels, and veterinary hospitals. Disease outbreaks involving only one species of infectious agent are possible, as seen in distemper outbreaks in susceptible populations [1]. Most commonly, however, infectious respiratory disease in dogs has a multifactorial etiology and is best described as canine infectious respiratory disease (CIRD) complex (also known as "kennel cough").

Viruses detected in dogs with CIRD include canine parainfluenza virus (CPIV) [2], canine adenovirus (CAV) type 2 [3] and canine herpesvirus [4]. Canine influenza virus, which recently has been detected in some parts of the United States, is likely to become part of the disease complex because it often causes mild respiratory disease characterized by nasal discharge and persistent cough [5].

Bacteria are important in CIRD as primary pathogens and as a cause of secondary infections. *Bordetella bronchiseptica* is the bacterium most frequently associated with CIRD [6], but mycoplasmas, particularly *Mycoplasma cynos*, have also been linked to the disease [6,7]. *Streptococcus equi* subsp. *zooepidemicus* has been isolated from severe cases of respiratory disease that were frequently fatal [8]. Vaccines have been developed for protection against several canine respiratory pathogens. Combination vaccines routinely contain canine distemper virus and CAV-1 or CAV-2. CAV vaccines confer cross-protection against type 1 (the cause of canine infectious hepatitis) and type 2 (associated with respiratory disease). CPIV is also included in several multivalent vaccines, or it is available in combination with *B bronchiseptica* as a "kennel cough vaccine."

This work was supported by Battersea Dogs and Cats Home and The Guide Dogs for the Blind Association.

*Corresponding author. E-mail address: kerles@rvc.ac.uk (K. Erles).

0195-5616/08/$ – see front matter
doi:10.1016/j.cvsm.2008.02.008

These are generally formulated for intranasal administration to provide a fast mucosal immune response. Despite the widespread use of vaccines, CIRD is an ongoing problem in many kennels. Possible causes are a lack of protection because of antigenic variants, the presence of known infectious agents for which vaccines have not yet been developed (eg, mycoplasmas), and the presence of novel infectious agents.

ORIGINS OF CANINE RESPIRATORY CORONAVIRUS

Canine respiratory coronavirus (CRCoV) was first detected in 2003 in dogs housed at a UK rehoming center [9]. The center had a high turnover of dogs and was reporting problems with enzootic respiratory disease despite regular vaccination. An investigation into pathogens associated with CIRD in this population led to the detection of a coronavirus in tracheal and lung samples by reverse transcriptase polymerase chain reaction (RT-PCR).

Coronaviruses are large enveloped viruses containing a positive-sense single-stranded RNA genome. The structural proteins located in the viral envelope include the spike protein (S), the membrane protein (M), and the small membrane protein (E). Initial sequence analysis of CRCoV showed a high similarity to bovine coronavirus (BCoV) and human coronavirus OC43 (96% amino acid identity with BCoV in the variable spike protein).

Coronaviruses had been described before in dogs with gastroenteritis [10]; however, it was shown that CRCoV was distinct from the previously known canine coronavirus (CCoV). The virus showed only 69% nucleotide identity in the highly conserved polymerase region and only 21% amino acid sequence identity in the spike protein, indicating that CRCoV was a novel coronavirus of dogs.

Members of the family Coronaviridae are separated into groups according to their genetic similarities [11]. Most members of group 2 of coronaviruses contain an additional gene coding for a surface hemagglutinin-esterase protein. This gene was found to be present in CRCoV, confirming its place in group 2 together with its closest relative, BCoV (Fig. 1). CCoV, in contrast is a member of group 1, which includes feline coronavirus and porcine transmissible gastroenteritis among others.

Currently, the oldest samples that tested positive for CRCoV are canine lung samples collected in Canada in 1996 [12]. One of the reasons precluding earlier discovery of CRCoV may be its poor growth in cell culture and the requirement for specific host cells. The close genetic relation to BCoV throughout the CRCoV genome indicates that the virus was probably transmitted to dogs from cattle [13]. Interestingly, it has recently been shown that human coronavirus OC43 also may have emerged after viral transmission from cattle to people [14].

EPIDEMIOLOGY

Coronaviruses are a cause of respiratory disease in many species, including human beings, poultry, and cattle [15–20]. The presence of CRCoV in dogs was first described in a large study of dogs with CIRD [9]. In this investigation,

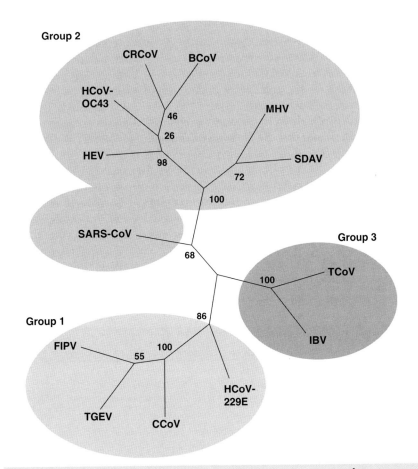

Fig. 1. Phylogenetic tree based on the partial polymerase gene sequence of coronaviruses. Gray shaded areas show the separation into groups 1 to 3. CRCoV is situated in group 2 with the most closely related species, BCoV, human coronavirus strain OC43 (HCoV-OC43), and porcine hemagglutinating encephalomyelitis virus (HEV), in addition to murine hepatitis virus (MHV) and rat sialodacryoadenitis virus (SDAV). Group 1 contains enteric CCoV, porcine transmissible gastroenteritis virus (TGEV), feline infectious peritonitis virus (FIPV), and human coronavirus strain 229E (HCoV-229E). Group 3 contains the avian coronaviruses infectious bronchitis virus (IBV) and turkey coronavirus (TCoV). Severe acute respiratory syndrome (SARS) coronavirus is currently classified as part of group 2 but may be reclassified as a new group 4 with related bat coronaviruses.

performed at a shelter, clinical signs were graded by veterinary clinicians into (1) no signs of respiratory disease; (2) mild cough; (3) mild cough and nasal discharge; (4) cough, nasal discharge, and inappetence; and (5) severe respiratory disease with evidence of bronchopneumonia. Because of a small number of samples in grade 4, grades 3 and 4 were merged and referred to as "moderate respiratory disease." CRCoV was most frequently detected in the trachea of dogs with mild clinical signs (grade 2). It was less frequently recovered from dogs with moderate or severe clinical signs or from dogs without clinical signs at the time of sampling. CRCoV was also detected in the lung, albeit less frequently. Table 1 summarizes the detection of CRCoV in clinical samples from dogs.

After 3 weeks of stay at a shelter, almost 100% of dogs tested positive for antibodies to CRCoV compared with 30% on the day of entry, indicating that the virus was highly prevalent in the population and was easily transmitted. It was also found that the presence of antibodies to CRCoV on the day of entry led to a significantly reduced risk for contracting CIRD, supporting the hypothesis that CRCoV played a role in the etiology of the disease [9].

After this initial investigation, CRCoV was also detected in two UK training kennels for working dogs [21]. Serum samples had been collected during two outbreaks of respiratory disease at one of the kennels and 4 weeks after. Almost all dogs housed at the kennel showed seroconversion to CRCoV after the outbreaks. Moreover, CRCoV was detected by PCR in two oropharyngeal swabs taken from dogs with clinical respiratory disease. Not all dogs that developed antibodies to CRCoV also showed signs of CIRD; nevertheless, this was the second study associating CRCoV with respiratory disease in dogs.

Table 1
Detection of canine respiratory coronavirus in clinical samples from dogs

Sample type	Clinical signs or histopathologic diagnosis	No. CRCoV-positive samples out of total no. samples (%)	Reference
Trachea	None	11 of 42 (26.1)	[9]
	Mild respiratory disease[a]	10 of 18 (55.6)	[9]
	Moderate respiratory disease	9 of 46 (19.6)	[9]
	Severe respiratory disease	2 of 13 (15.4)	[9]
Lung	None	8 of 42 (19)	[9]
	Mild respiratory disease	4 of 18 (22.2)	[9]
	Moderate respiratory disease	8 of 46 (17.4)	[9]
	Severe respiratory disease	0 of 13	[9]
Lung	Severe gastroenteritis[b]	1 of 109 (0.92)	[26]
Lung	Bronchitis/bronchiolitis	2 of 126 (1.6)	[12]
Oropharyngeal swab	Mild respiratory disease	2 of 64 (3.1)	[21]
Oropharyngeal swab	None	1 of 64 (1.6)	[21]
Oral swab	Cough	1 of 10 (10)	[23]
Oral swab	None	1 of 10 (10)	[23]
Nasal swab	Cough and nasal discharge	1 of 59 (1.7)	[22]
Rectal swab	Gastroenteritis[c]	1 of 65 (1.5)	[22]

[a]Criteria for grading into mild, moderate, and severe respiratory disease are explained in the section on epidemiology.
[b]Evidence of bronchopneumonia at postmortem examination, canine parvovirus, and CCoV also detected.
[c]CCoV and CPIV also detected.

Two further studies identified CRCoV in nasal and oral swabs from dogs in Japan that had respiratory disease [22,23]. An analysis of 126 archival tissue blocks of cases of respiratory disease identified two CRCoV-positive samples by immunohistochemistry. Both were from dogs with bronchitis and bronchiolitis, and CRCoV antigen was found to be present in respiratory columnar epithelial cells. One of those dogs was also positive for canine distemper virus [12]. The detection rate of CRCoV in the archival study may seem quite low; however, the tissue samples were mostly derived from dogs with severe respiratory disease with a fatal outcome, whereas CRCoV has mostly been associated with mild respiratory disease so far.

Serologic studies to determine the prevalence of antibodies to CRCoV have been performed to date for the United Kingdom, Republic of Ireland, Italy, United States, Canada, and Japan. The highest seroprevalence was detected in Canada (59.1% of sera tested were found to be positive) and the United States (54.7% of sera tested were found to be positive). Samples from the United States had been collected from 33 states, and positive samples were identified in 29 [24]. In those states that allowed a meaningful interpretation of seroprevalence (more than 10 samples), the prevalence ranged from 31.3% (Maine) to 87.5% (Kentucky). The prevalence in the United Kingdom and the Republic of Ireland was lower, with 36% and 30.3%, respectively [24]. Two studies performed in Italy showed seroprevalence ranging from 20% to 32.5% [25,26]. The lowest seroprevalence was detected in Japan, with 17.8% [23]. Further data are not yet available, but it is likely that CRCoV is present throughout the United States and in other European countries.

Although CRCoV was detected throughout the year in a kennel with enzootic CIRD, another study reported a seasonal occurrence of the virus in the winter months. No seroconversions to CRCoV and few cases of respiratory disease were recorded in the summer months [21]. A similar seasonality has been reported for human coronaviruses involved in the common cold [27].

CRCoV infections can occur in dogs of all ages. Dogs younger than 1 year of age were significantly more likely to be seronegative than older dogs, however [24,25]. This is in contrast to the prevalence of enteric CCoV, which is frequently found in dogs younger than 1 year of age [10]. This may reflect different patterns of transmission of the two viruses. The seroprevalence of CRCoV was increasing after the age of 1 year for all studies and then reached a plateau between the ages of 2 and approximately 8 years. This is probably a consequence of the greater probability of exposure to the virus with increasing contact with other dogs. It is not certain how long CRCoV antibody levels in dogs remain stable after infection. One study showed a twofold decrease in antibody titers in 6 of 14 dogs tested and a fourfold decrease in 4 dogs in less than 1 year [21]. Because these were naturally occurring infections, it is not known if the antibody response measured reflected primary or repeated infections. The viral dose encountered by dogs would also influence the level and duration of the antibody response.

The rapid spread of CRCoV through kenneled populations indicates that the virus is highly contagious. This, in conjunction with the predominant detection of CRCoV in respiratory samples, suggests that it is mostly spread by means of respiratory secretions. CRCoV probably enters the respiratory tract by inhalation of droplets or contact with secretions and contaminated surfaces.

PATHOGENESIS AND CLINICAL SIGNS

It is not possible to discuss the pathogenesis and clinical signs associated with CRCoV without considering the CIRD complex as a whole. CRCoV has been detected in several studies in dogs with respiratory disease. In most of these cases, however, other respiratory pathogens were also present. In two detailed studies into the causes of CIRD in which evidence of CRCoV was reported, the dogs presented with the typical signs of a dry cough and nasal discharge [21,28]. Concurrent infections were most frequently caused by CPIV and *B bronchiseptica*.

CRCoV has also been detected in dogs that have nonrespiratory disease. It was detected in the lung, spleen, mesenteric lymph nodes, and intestines of a dog that had died from hemorrhagic gastroenteritis [26]. The dog also tested positive for canine parvovirus type 2 and CCoV. Similarly, CRCoV was detected in a rectal swab from a dog with vomiting and diarrhea, which was also positive for CCoV and CPIV [22]. In both cases, the concurrent infections with canine parvovirus or CCoV are likely to have been the cause of the clinical signs. Studies of the tissue distribution of CRCoV in 10 naturally infected dogs showed that CRCoV was most frequently detected in the nasal cavity, nasal tonsil, and trachea and less frequently in the lung, bronchial lymph nodes, and palatine tonsil. It was also detected in samples from the spleen, mesenteric lymph nodes, and colon but not in the enteric content (K. Erles, unpublished data, 2004). The tissue tropism of CRCoV therefore seems not to be exclusively respiratory, and fecal-oral transmission of CRCoV may be possible.

CRCoV may show a dual tropism, similar to BCoV, but the ability of the virus to replicate in the epithelium of the gastrointestinal tract and the clinical consequences need further investigation.

Experimental studies using CRCoV have not been reported to date. A study using BCoV showed that dogs became infected and transmitted the virus to contact dogs. BCoV was detected in rectal and oral swabs, and the dogs developed neutralizing antibodies to the virus [29]. The dogs did not develop fever or any clinical signs of respiratory or gastrointestinal disease. Despite their high similarity, BCoV may be less pathogenic in dogs compared with CRCoV. Furthermore, the etiology of CIRD has been shown to involve multiple pathogens. Viral infections can aid the entry of other pathogens by facilitating their attachment or by inhibition of the mucociliary clearance. Many pathogens known to be involved in the CIRD complex have also been found in dogs without clinical signs, including CPIV and *B bronchiseptica* [28,30]. When assessing the pathogenesis of complex diseases, it is important to consider the possible interaction of pathogens during coinfections and contributing factors, such as stress.

DIAGNOSIS

Because of the involvement of multiple pathogens in the etiology of CIRD, it is not possible to diagnose CRCoV solely by clinical signs. The most suitable test to diagnose CRCoV in respiratory samples is nested RT-PCR based on the spike glycoprotein gene [9] or the hemagglutinin-esterase gene [22]. This test has a high sensitivity, which is particularly useful when analyzing samples with a potentially low number of cells, such as oropharyngeal or nasal swabs. Both PCR methods are specific for CRCoV and do not detect enteric CCoV. Because the virus was found most frequently in the nasal cavity, nasal swabs are suitable diagnostic samples. CRCoV has also been detected in oral swabs, and, furthermore, nasal or tracheal washes are likely to yield CRCoV during an active infection. If postmortem samples are available, nasal cavity, nasal tonsil, trachea, and lung samples should be collected for analysis.

Isolation of CRCoV in cell culture has been achieved; however, it is not recommended to use virus isolation alone to diagnose CRCoV. To date, isolation of CRCoV has only succeeded on the human rectal tumor cell line HRT-18 and its clone HRT-18G [13]. Even on HRT-18 cells, the isolation of CRCoV from RT-PCR–positive samples is often unsuccessful [22,23,26]. The only isolate of CRCoV that has so far been studied in detail did not produce a cytopathic effect on HRT-18 cells, and infection had to be confirmed by using immunofluorescence or PCR. Supernatants from infected cell cultures were found to agglutinate chicken erythrocytes at 4°C [13]. Hemagglutination assays may aid in detection of CRCoV-infected cell cultures if isolation is attempted.

CRCoV has also been detected by immunohistochemistry on formalin-fixed tissues using an antibody directed against BCoV [12]. The sensitivity of immunohistochemistry in comparison to PCR has not been evaluated; however, this method is useful for testing archival respiratory samples.

Serology is a valuable tool for the detection of CRCoV infections if paired serum samples are collected during an outbreak of respiratory disease and at least 2 to 3 weeks afterward. The high similarity of CRCoV and BCoV allows the use of BCoV antigens to test canine sera by ELISA [9,26]. Similarly, BCoV has been used instead of CRCoV in serum neutralization tests [23]. A hemagglutination inhibition test based on BCoV has also been evaluated but was assessed as having poor sensitivity and specificity compared with an ELISA based on BCoV [26].

An ELISA assay using CRCoV antigen was found to have slightly higher sensitivity and specificity compared with an assay based on BCoV; however, overall, the agreement between the two ELISA tests was high [24]. Antibodies to CRCoV have also been detected by using an immunofluorescence assay on CRCoV-infected HRT-18 cells [24].

Specific tests for CRCoV are becoming increasingly available; however, most assays offered for the detection of coronaviruses in dogs are specific for enteric CCoV. Antibodies to CRCoV do not cross-react with enteric CCoV. It is important to use an assay capable of detecting antibodies to CRCoV or related group 2 coronaviruses, such as BCoV. Consequently, the requirement for CRCoV detection should be discussed with the diagnostic laboratory before submitting samples for RT-PCR, virus isolation, or serology.

TREATMENT

There is no specific treatment for infections caused by CRCoV. As for other causes of CIRD, patient care should focus on the prevention and treatment of bacterial infections. Although many pathogens involved in CIRD are reported to be associated with mild clinical disease, it is important to bear in mind that mixed infections can potentially be much more severe. Patients should be monitored, because the condition may rapidly worsen. Severe cases of CIRD with sudden death have been reported after infections with *Streptococcus equi* subsp. *zooepidemicus* [8].

PREVENTION

To date, no vaccines against CRCoV are available. Vaccines against CCoV are unlikely to protect against infection with CRCoV because of a low similarity in the spike proteins that are the major immunogenic proteins of coronaviruses. Vaccines against other respiratory pathogens may not prevent CIRD, particularly in large populations because of the presence of other infectious agents. Nevertheless, they have the potential to reduce the number of circulating pathogens if given to all dogs on entry. Vaccines against canine distemper virus and CAV are widely used, and this may account for the inability to identify either virus in a population with enzootic CIRD [28].

Although no specific tests have been performed to determine the stability of CRCoV in the environment, other coronaviruses have been reported to remain infectious in respiratory secretions for more than 7 days [31]. Thorough cleaning and disinfection of kennels after outbreaks of respiratory disease are therefore required. Coronaviruses are inactivated by disinfectants commonly used for surface disinfection in kennels and veterinary practices. The role of fecal shedding and the potential transmission of CRCoV among dogs sharing common facilities, such as outdoor runs, have yet to be resolved. Other generally recommended measures, such as washing one's hands after handling animals with respiratory disease should also help to reduce the spread of the virus. CRCoV has been detected in dogs up to 4 weeks after entry into a kennel. Because the time of infection in those naturally occurring cases is not known, it is unclear how long CRCoV is being shed. After experimental infection of dogs with BCoV, the virus was detected in a rectal swab after 11 days [29]. Quarantine of newly arriving dogs, if feasible in training kennels or shelters, should therefore last for at least 2 weeks.

PRESENCE OF GROUP 1 CANINE CORONAVIRUS IN THE RESPIRATORY TRACT

Group 1 CCoVs, referred to in this article as CCoVs, have previously been associated with mild gastroenteritis. According to their similarity to feline coronaviruses, they are divided into type I (related to feline coronavirus type I) or type II (related to feline coronavirus type II) [32]. Although CCoV has been isolated from the lung after experimental infections [33], it was generally considered to be restricted to the gastrointestinal tract during naturally occurring infection. Recently, an outbreak of a systemic fatal disease was described from which a type II CCoV was isolated [34]. Although the dogs presented with vomiting, diarrhea, and neurologic signs, postmortem examination also revealed bronchopneumonia. CCoV was detected in internal organs, including the lung, kidney, and brain. Sequence analysis of the CCoV isolate identified a mutation in open reading frame 3b, leading to a truncated nonstructural protein. It is not clear if this mutation is responsible for the extended tropism of this isolate [35]. Further studies are required to determine the presence of type II CCoVs in cases of severe systemic disease and in cases of respiratory disease.

SUMMARY

CRCoV is a novel coronavirus of dogs distinct from CCoV. It is present in North America, Europe, and Japan. CRCoV is frequently detected in dogs with clinical respiratory signs and may contribute to the CIRD complex. Increased awareness of the existence of CRCoV and the development of routinely available diagnostic tests should enhance our knowledge of the presence of CRCoV in canine populations with and without respiratory disease. It is recommended to use PCR methods or serology on paired serum samples to diagnose CRCoV infections, because the sensitivity of virus isolation is low. Identification of causative agents during outbreaks of respiratory disease in canine populations ought to be performed more frequently. This would help to determine the importance of individual viruses and bacteria, not only in the investigated population but in the CIRD complex as a whole. The etiology of CIRD is multifactorial and is likely to change continuously, because some pathogens are controlled by vaccination, although other infectious agents emerge to take their place.

References

[1] Norris JM, Krockenberger MB, Baird AA, et al. Canine distemper: re-emergence of an old enemy. Aust Vet J 2006;84:362–3.
[2] Appel MJ, Percy DH. SV-5-like parainfluenza virus in dogs. J Am Vet Med Assoc 1970;156: 1778–81.
[3] Ditchfield J, Macpherson LW, Zbitnew A. Association of canine adenovirus (Toronto A 26/61) with an outbreak of laryngotracheitis ("kennel cough"): a preliminary report. Can Vet J 1962;3:238–47.
[4] Karpas A, King NW, Garcia FG, et al. Canine tracheobronchitis: isolation and characterization of the agent with experimental reproduction of the disease. Proc Soc Exp Biol Med 1968;127:45–52.
[5] Crawford PC, Dubovi EJ, Castleman WL, et al. Transmission of equine influenza virus to dogs. Science 2005;310:482–5.
[6] Bemis DA. Bordetella and mycoplasma respiratory infections in dogs and cats. Vet Clin North Am Small Anim Pract 1992;22:1173–86.
[7] Chalker VJ, Owen WM, Paterson C, et al. Mycoplasmas associated with canine infectious respiratory disease. Microbiology 2004;150:3491–7.

[8] Chalker VJ, Brooks HW, Brownlie J. The association of streptococcus equi subsp. zooepide-
     micus with canine infectious respiratory disease. Vet Microbiol 2003;95:149–56.
[9] Erles K, Toomey C, Brooks HW, et al. Detection of a group 2 coronavirus in dogs with canine
     infectious respiratory disease. Virology 2003;310:216–23.
[10] Tennant BJ, Gaskell RM, Jones RC, et al. Studies on the epizootiology of canine coronavirus.
     Vet Rec 1993;132:7–11.
[11] Weiss SR, Navas-Martin S. Coronavirus pathogenesis and the emerging pathogen severe
     acute respiratory syndrome coronavirus. Microbiol Mol Biol Rev 2005;69:635–64.
[12] Ellis JA, McLean N, Hupaelo R, et al. Detection of coronavirus in cases of tracheobronchitis
     in dogs: a retrospective study from 1971 to 2003. Can Vet J 2005;46:447–8.
[13] Erles K, Shiu K-B, Brownlie J. Isolation and sequence analysis of canine respiratory corona-
     virus. Virus Res 2007;124:78–87.
[14] Vijgen L, Keyaerts E, Moes E, et al. Complete genomic sequence of human coronavirus
     OC43: molecular clock analysis suggests a relatively recent zoonotic coronavirus transmis-
     sion event. J Virol 2005;79:1595–604.
[15] Peiris JS, Lai ST, Poon LL, et al. Coronavirus as a possible cause of severe acute respiratory
     syndrome. Lancet 2003;361:1319–25.
[16] Makela MJ, Puhakka T, Ruuskanen O, et al. Viruses and bacteria in the etiology of the com-
     mon cold. J Clin Microbiol 1998;36:539–42.
[17] van der Hoek L, Pyrc K, Jebbink MF, et al. Identification of a new human coronavirus. Nat
     Med 2004;10:368–73.
[18] Woo PCY, Lau SKP, Chu C-M, et al. Characterization and complete genome sequence of
     a novel coronavirus, coronavirus HKU1, from patients with pneumonia. J Virol 2005;79:
     884–95.
[19] Cavanagh D. Coronavirus avian infectious bronchitis virus. Vet Res 2007;38:281–97.
[20] Storz J, Lin X, Purdy CW, et al. Coronavirus and Pasteurella infections in bovine shipping
     fever pneumonia and Evans' criteria for causation. J Clin Microbiol 2000;38:3291–8.
[21] Erles K, Brownlie J. Investigation into the causes of canine infectious respiratory disease: an-
     tibody responses to canine respiratory coronavirus and canine herpesvirus in two kennelled
     dog populations. Arch Virol 2005;150:1493–504.
[22] Yachi A, Mochizuki M. Survey of dogs in Japan for group 2 canine coronavirus infection.
     J Clin Microbiol 2006;44:2615–8.
[23] Kaneshima T, Hohdatsu T, Satoh K, et al. The prevalence of a group 2 coronavirus in dogs in
     Japan. J Vet Med Sci 2006;68:21–5.
[24] Priestnall SL, Brownlie J, Dubovi EJ, et al. Serological prevalence of canine respiratory
     coronavirus. Vet Microbiol 2006;115:43–53.
[25] Priestnall SL, Pratelli A, Brownlie J, et al. Serological prevalence of canine respiratory coro-
     navirus in southern Italy and epidemiological relationship with canine enteric coronavirus.
     J Vet Diagn Invest 2007;19:176–80.
[26] Decaro N, Desario C, Elia G, et al. Serological and molecular evidence that canine respi-
     ratory coronavirus is circulating in Italy. Vet Microbiol 2007;121:225–30.
[27] Isaacs D, Flowers D, Clarke JR, et al. Epidemiology of coronavirus respiratory infections.
     Arch Dis Child 1983;58:500–3.
[28] Erles K, Dubovi EJ, Brooks HW, et al. Longitudinal study of viruses associated with canine
     infectious respiratory disease. J Clin Microbiol 2004;42:4524–9.
[29] Kaneshima T, Hohdatsu T, Hagino R, et al. The infectivity and pathogenicity of a group 2
     bovine coronavirus in pups. J Vet Med Sci 2007;69:301–3.
[30] Chalker VJ, Toomey C, Opperman S, et al. Respiratory disease in kennelled dogs: sero-
     logical responses to bordetella bronchiseptica lipopolysaccharide do not correlate with
     bacterial isolation or clinical respiratory symptoms. Clin Diagn Lab Immunol 2003;10:
     352–6.
[31] Lai MYY, Cheng PKC, Lim WWL. Survival of severe acute respiratory syndrome coronavirus.
     Clin Infect Dis 2005;41:e67–71.

[32] Pratelli A, Martella V, Decaro N, et al. Genetic diversity of a canine coronavirus detected in pups with diarrhoea in Italy. J Virol Methods 2003;110:9–17.
[33] Tennant BJ, Gaskell RM, Kelly DF, et al. Canine coronavirus infection in the dog following oronasal inoculation. Res Vet Sci 1991;51:11–8.
[34] Buonavoglia C, Decaro N, Martella V, et al. Canine coronavirus highly pathogenic for dogs. Emerg Infect Dis 2006;12:492–4.
[35] Decaro N, Martella V, Elia G, et al. Molecular characterisation of the virulent canine coronavirus CB/05 strain. Virus Res 2007;125:54–60.

Vet Clin Small Anim 38 (2008) 827–835

VETERINARY CLINICS
SMALL ANIMAL PRACTICE

Canine Influenza

Edward J. Dubovi, PhD[a],*, Bradley L. Njaa, DVM, MVSc[b]

[a]Department of Population Medicine and Diagnostic Sciences, Animal Health Diagnostic Center, College of Veterinary Medicine, Cornell University, Ithaca, NY 14853, USA
[b]Department of Veterinary Pathobiology, Center for Veterinary Health Sciences, Oklahoma State University, 226 McElroy Hall, Stillwater, OK 74078, USA

When beginning a discussion about "canine influenza" one must make a clear distinction between influenza virus infections in canids and an infection of canids by a virus with the characteristics of canine influenza virus (CIV). Reports of experimental and natural infections of canids by human strains of influenza have existed for years [1,2], but no data have indicated a role of canids in human influenza virus infections and there has been no evidence of clinical disease in the infected animals. More recently, field and experimental data show that canids are susceptible to the Asian H5N1 viruses; however, again, no maintenance of the virus in the canine population has been demonstrated [3–7]. These instances simply show that canids can be infected with influenza viruses, but transmission within the canine population was not identified.

In 2004, the isolation of an influenza virus from racing greyhounds changed the point of reference for discussions about influenza virus in dogs [8]. A virus isolated from greyhounds did not have its origin in a previously described human influenza virus but came from a virus with an equine history. More significantly, evidence emerged to indicate that the virus was capable of transmission from dog to dog. This virus is now referred to as CIV and is the focus of this review. Because the history of CIV is relatively short, the impact of this virus on canine health is yet to be determined.

HISTORICAL ASPECTS

The greyhound racing industry had been plagued by significant respiratory problems in the dogs associated with the tracks for several years. Tests for the known pathogens linked to respiratory disease in dogs failed to identify the cause of the recurring problems. In January of 2004, another outbreak of respiratory disease occurred at a racetrack in Florida [8]. Of the 22 animals involved, 8 died acutely with extensive hemorrhage in the lungs. From one of these fatalities, a virus was isolated that had not been found previously in dogs. Subsequent characterization of the virus indicated that it was a group

*Corresponding author. E-mail address: ejd5@cornell.edu (E.J. Dubovi).

0195-5616/08/$ – see front matter
doi:10.1016/j.cvsm.2008.03.004

A influenza virus linked to an equine lineage (H3N8). At the time, it was not known if this was simply another influenza virus in a dog or if it was an influenza virus that had established itself in the canine population. Serologic data obtained using canine/FL/04 as a test antigen showed that infections with influenza virus were not confined to a single racetrack but were present in other locations in Florida.

The extent of the infections in greyhounds was shown in 2004 to 2005 by two lines of evidence. Respiratory disease outbreaks occurred during this period at racetracks in at least 13 states representing more than 20,000 dogs [8]. Sera collected from 5 of these states showed that high percentages of dogs were seropositive for CIV, with numerous cases of seroconversion to CIV across the respiratory outbreaks. In July 2004, a second influenza virus was isolated from the lungs of a greyhound that died at a track in Texas (canine/TX/04). Sequence analysis of the virus showed at least 99% nucleotide homology with canine/FL/04 and confirmed the H3N8 equine link to CIV [8]. In April 2005, a respiratory disease outbreak occurred at an Iowa racetrack resulting in essentially a 100% morbidity rate, but less than 5% of dogs died with signs similar to those that died in the January 2004 outbreak in Florida [9]. Two of four animals examined were positive for influenza virus by polymerase chain reaction (PCR) assay and immunohistochemistry. Sequence analysis showed the link to recent H3N8 equine viruses, and subsequent comparisons among the Florida, Texas, and canine/IA/05 isolates showed a common lineage [10]. In aggregate, these data established the fact of widespread infections in greyhounds in the racing industry with CIV and made it virtually impossible to deny the existence of an influenza virus in canids capable of horizontal transmission among the dogs.

As indicated previously, the problem of respiratory outbreaks in the greyhound racing industry had been evident for several years. In light of this new evidence, archived samples from outbreaks previous to January 2004 were re-evaluated. Examination of tissues from a dog that died in March 2003 yielded another influenza virus isolate (canine/Fl/03) that had high sequence homology to canine/FL/04 [8]. Of a limited number of sera available from previous outbreaks, one of four sera from 2000 was positive for antibodies to CIV. Thus, CIV was in the greyhound population for at least several years before its initial detection in 2004.

Although the finding of CIV in greyhounds was a significant discovery, the focus of the investigation quickly became the nonracing canine population. Serologic data from sera collected from shelters and pet clinics in Florida and New York demonstrated the presence of CIV in the pet population [8]. Isolation of CIV from pet dogs in Florida and New York in 2005 established conclusive proof that CIV infections were not restricted to greyhounds under racing conditions and that all breeds seemed to be fully susceptible to CIV (E.J. Dubovi, unpublished data, 2006) [10]. The data from New York established CIV as the cause of a major epizootic in the New York City area in the summer of 2005 and clearly established that CIV had moved from the pet population of Florida to the Northeast by the middle of 2005.

The movement of CIV in the canine pet population has been unpredictable, as is the movement of dogs by owners and the various rescue organizations. The Florida–New York area link is understandable, given the large number of individuals that move between these locations in the spring and fall. Serologic data on CIV began to be collected in the fall of 2005 at the Animal Health Diagnostic Center (AHDC) at Cornell University, Ithaca, New York from submissions throughout the country [11]. Initial results clearly showed the presence of CIV in Florida and the New York City area (New York, New Jersey, and Connecticut). A few positive animals were detected in Arizona and California at this time. Because there were no isolates of CIV from this region, one could not tell whether this was from CIV (greyhound track in Arizona) or simply another type A influenza virus in dogs. Seroconversions to CIV were identified in the Washington, DC area in private practices and in a shelter in Delaware. Inexplicably, the virus seems to have disappeared from these areas, because no further virus activity has been noted to date.

In December 2006, reports began to surface of unusual respiratory outbreaks in kennels and shelters in the Denver, Colorado area. In January 2006, serologic data showed the presence of CIV in the Colorado area and subsequent testing detected CIV by PCR assay and by virus isolation (canine/CO/06) (E.J. Dubovi, unpublished data, 2006). The virus is now enzootic in Colorado, as it is in Florida and New York. Virus was detected in Wyoming and San Diego, California in May 2005. The San Diego outbreak was linked to the movement of a dog from Colorado to southern California. Strict quarantine of the affected kennel seemed to prevent spread to other locations in the San Diego area. Seroconversions were also noted in Utah in August 2006, presumably as an offshoot of the Colorado epizootic.

Other outbreaks, as defined by isolation of CIV, were in Kentucky (September 2006), western Pennsylvania (January 2007), eastern Pennsylvania (July 2007), and Los Angeles, California (July 2007) (E.J. Dubovi, unpublished data, 2007). These were in addition to the ongoing presence of the virus in Florida, the New York City area, and Colorado. All other areas of the country seem to be unaffected by CIV as of March 2008 based on the lack of viral isolates and the lack of positive sera (E.J. Dubovi and P.D. Kirkland, unpublished data, 2008). The somewhat sporadic movement of the virus certainly is related to movement of dogs but also to the exposure and minimal movement controls of susceptible dogs in new locations. As a case in point, a dog was moved from New York City to Ithaca, New York at the end of December 2006. It developed respiratory signs on arrival and exposed other dogs in the kennel. CIV was diagnosed based on serology, and a voluntary quarantine was placed on the kennel. Others in the group became infected as determined by serology, but the virus did not spread in the community because of the movement restrictions and lack of contact with other susceptible dogs.

The isolation of CIV in 2004 initiated studies in other countries to determine the presence of influenza virus in dogs. The only published reports to date have come from England. In a retrospective study, researchers at the Animal Health

Trust detected equine influenza virus as the cause of a respiratory outbreak in a quarry hound kennel in 2002, but there was no evidence for ongoing transmission [12]. Limited sequence analysis of nucleic acid recovered from fixed tissues from a dog that died confirmed the equine origin of the H3 virus linked to the outbreak. No data were presented to show that CIV was involved in the outbreak, however. In a second report, serologic evidence was presented suggesting that foxhounds became infected with a newly introduced H3N8 virus in the spring of 2003 [13]. Again, there was no evidence of horizontal transmission or a link to CIV. The epizootic of H3N8 in equids in Australia in 2007 also resulted in infected dogs (P.D. Kirkland, personal communication, 2008). Animals in contact with horses have shown seroconversion, and although clinical signs were noted in a moderate proportion, there was no evidence of horizontal transmission among the dogs. These cases seem to be equine influenza virus in dogs and not CIV infections.

CLINICAL PRESENTATIONS

The challenge in dealing with CIV is that like many respiratory pathogens, the signs associated with the infection overlap with other agents. In most cases, a clinician would be hard pressed to distinguish a CIV infection from those agents that cause "kennel cough." Virtually all CIV cases in the canine pet population investigated at the AHDC are linked to shelters, boarding kennels, or "doggie" day care centers, a feature not different from kennel cough. Distinctive of CIV infections is the degree of morbidity within the facility. For kennel cough, a few dogs exhibit clinical signs, because prior exposure and vaccination reduce the attack rate. For CIV, virtually all dogs are susceptible regardless of age, and attack rates of 60% to 80% are not unusual. The presence of CIV in the New York City area was identified by the observations of an astute practitioner who noted that the normal fewer than 5 cases of kennel cough per month had exploded to more than 100. This individual had used "syndromic surveillance" to detect the presence of a new pathogen in his practice area.

The signs associated with most CIV infections are not pathognomonic. The onset of clinical signs is less than 5 days after infection with 2 to 3 days being most common. The presenting signs are somewhat related to the time from infection to the date of the examination (E.J. Dubovi, unpublished data, 2006). Virtually all dogs are described as being lethargic and anorexic with a nasal discharge. Initially, the nasal discharge is clear, but it quickly becomes mucopurulent. Most dogs early in the infection show a low-grade fever. A persistent cough that is usually dry and nonproductive develops and may last for several weeks. Many dogs are diagnosed as having pneumonia, bronchopneumonia, or abnormal lung sounds. In most instances, the serious lung involvement is attributable to the secondary bacteria or mycoplasma infections that are manifest with compromised lung defenses. A mortality rate attributable directly to CIV infection is difficult to determine, given the high frequency of coinfection by other respiratory agents. Fortunately, the more severe form of the disease (hemorrhagic pneumonia), as seen in the Florida greyhounds, is not manifest in the pet population [8]. The severe hemorrhagic pneumonia reported in racing greyhounds in an Iowa outbreak was complicated by the concurrent coinfection of CIV and *Streptococcus equi* subsp. *zooepidemicus* [9]. Peracute deaths are rarely reported, and deaths associated with CIV tend to be associated with longer treatment periods.

PATHOLOGIC FINDINGS

Limited information exists about the lesions associated with CIV infection in dogs. Early reports divided the disease syndromes into two distinct clinical entities [8]. The more common syndrome is the mild disease, which rarely leads to death and seems similar to episodes of kennel cough. Based on some experimental infections in naive populations of puppies, cranioventral lung consolidation was rarely observed in infected dogs (B.L. Njaa, unpublished data, 2006). Bronchial lymph nodes were variably megalgic and edematous. Scattered through the more severely affected lungs were small focal areas of pulmonary hemorrhage. Severe hemorrhagic pneumonia was not seen in any of the experimentally infected dogs.

Gross lesions associated with the second less common but more severe syndrome were dramatic. In both published accounts, the lungs were reportedly dark red to black and moderately to markedly palpably firm [8,9] In addition, hemorrhages were evident in the mediastinum, and there was a hemorrhagic effusion in the pleural cavity [8].

Whether the severe hemorrhagic variant or the less severe disease form, histologic lesions documented from published accounts are similar. Alveolar septa are thickened because of edema and inflammatory cell infiltration with or without hemorrhage depending on the syndrome. Alveolar changes vary from localized areas of atelectasis, to aggregates of cellular debris, to infiltration by neutrophils and macrophages. In the severe hemorrhagic syndrome, there are large amounts of hemorrhagic exudate within the interstitium in addition to the airway and alveolar lumens. Vasculitis and intravascular thrombi are also seen in the severe hemorrhagic pneumonic disease [8,9].

The trachea, bronchi, and bronchioles are similarly affected with loss of ciliated epithelial cells; attenuation of the remaining lining epithelial cells; infiltration of the propria-submucosa by mixtures of inflammatory cells that vary from predominant neutrophilic to pyogranulomatous to lymphoplasmacytic; exocytosis of variable mixtures of neutrophils, lymphocytes, and macrophages through the lining epithelium; and aggregates of sloughed epithelial cells mixed with degenerate and nondegenerate neutrophils and macrophages within airway lumens (B.L. Njaa, unpublished data, 2006) [8].

VIROLOGY

The sequence analysis of canine/FL/04 unequivocally established that CIV originated in the H3N8 equine lineage [8]. This cross-species transmission came about as a result of the entire H3N8 genome being represented in CIV without any genomic reassortment. Although the history of equine H3N8 begins in 1963, the CIV isolates of 2003 to 2005 are most closely matched to US equine isolates of 2003 [8,10]. Serologic data suggest that CIV was in the canine population before 2003, but representative equine or canine isolates from this earlier period are not available currently to establish the progenitor of CIV. The sequence of the HA gene of six canine isolates (2003–2005) was compared with several contemporary equine influenza viruses, and five amino acid differences were noted that distinguished the canine viruses from the equine viruses [8,10]. With respect to the HA0 protein, these changes and locations are: N54K, N83S, W222L, I328T, and N483T. Whether any of these changes are related to the ability of equine influenza virus to infect and be transmitted among canids is unknown at this time. There is also some suggestion that the canine isolates may be evolving into separate clades, but more of the later (2006–2008) isolates need to be sequenced to establish any patterns.

DIAGNOSTICS

As with any infectious disease, the keys to a successful diagnosis are to have basic knowledge of the infection parameters and to have reliable diagnostic tests with adequate sensitivity and specificity. For CIV, there is limited published information that directly relates to defining the optimum diagnostic testing. Optimal testing strategies may well come into conflict with the realities of the clinical setting. For antemortem testing, transtracheal washes (TTWs) are ideal samples for all respiratory agents. Few owners and practitioners are willing to perform this costly procedure if a swab is sufficient, however. At present, there are no published data on the comparison of TTWs and swabs for CIV diagnosis.

The initial report of CIV presented some data on the challenge of 4 dogs with the initial CIV isolate [8], and unpublished observations and a subsequent publication have greatly expanded on these initial observations (E.J. Dubovi, unpublished observations, 2006) [14]. A key question that needed to be answered was identification of the best sample to collect in a clinical setting to detect the presence of CIV. Initial sampling focused on pharyngeal swabs, and positive results were meager (E.J. Dubovi, unpublished observations, 2006). In a challenge study, 77 nasal and 77 pharyngeal swabs were collected over a 7-day period. CIV was detected from 72% of the nasal swabs and from only 32% of the pharyngeal swabs. These data focused all subsequent sampling at the AHDC on nasal swabs.

The challenge data also showed that the amount of virus shed was less than 5 $\log_{10}$ in the test samples, with peak infectious virus titers in the 2- to 5-day postinfection period. Infectious virus was not detectable in the 8- to 9-day postinfection period. Antibody titers detected by hemagglutination inhibition (HI) were detectable by 7 to 8 days after infection, with titers reaching 512 to 1024 by days 13 to 14 after infection (E.J. Dubovi, unpublished observations) [14]. These data clearly indicate that testing directly for the virus in a patient that has been showing clinical signs for more than 3 days (5–6 days after infection) are largely nonproductive.

Detection of a viral infection is generally done in one of four ways or in various combinations. Traditional methods include isolation of the virus. For influenza viruses, two systems are routinely used: embryonated eggs and MDCK cells with a protease overlay. At this point in time, it does not seem that one system is substantially better than the other. Isolates from single samples have been obtained in both systems, in cell culture but not eggs, and in eggs but not cell culture (E.J. Dubovi, unpublished observations, 2006). To maximize yield, both systems should be used. For the egg system, the samples should be blind-passed at least once, because H3 viruses do not grow as efficiently in this system as other influenza H types. Virus isolation for CIV is still a critical test to perform, because this is a new virus in an entirely susceptible population. The evolution of this virus is unpredictable, and monitoring of changes in the virus as it moves through the canine population is important in defining new tests and potentially new vaccines.

Influenza viruses are now easily detectable by various PCR tests. As with virus isolation, the timing and collection site of the sample are critical in determining the success of the test. At the AHDC at Cornell University, the sample routinely tested is a nasal swab with a collection time of not more than 3 to 4 days after the onset of symptoms. The target of the PCR assay can be the same matrix gene sequence that is used for avian influenza virus surveillance by the National Animal Health Laboratory Network. Although it would be possible to have an H3-specific PCR assay, the preferred method is to screen for the presence of any influenza virus in a clinical sample. If positive, one can then proceed to determine the H type directly or after isolation of the virus. In this manner, diagnostic laboratories are unlikely to miss influenza virus in dogs. Approximately 75% of PCR-positive samples under these test conditions yield a virus on isolation using the egg-cell culture procedures. In the case of postmortem tissues, there may be significantly more PCR-positive samples than virus isolation (VI)-positive samples because of the fact that death may have occurred when an immune response had developed and no infectious-free virus is present.

Antigen-capture ELISA tests have been used successfully to detect H3 viruses in horses, and use in dogs would be a logical extension. Unfortunately, testing in dogs has not been as successful as in horses. The reason for this may be the apparent low amount of virus shed by dogs. On an individual dog basis, the tests are not recommended, but in a kennel outbreak in which some dogs may be at the peak of virus shed, the testing may detect an outbreak.

Serologic testing is still an important component of a diagnostic workup. For dogs that have been coughing for longer than 5 days before they are seen by a practitioner, the only testing that may define CIV status is antibody detection. Although microneutralization tests can be done [8], this is too cumbersome for routine testing. The standard HI test with a slight modification is more than adequate for detecting antibodies to CIV [8,15]. For CIV, chicken red blood

cells are replaced with tom turkey red blood cells because H3 viruses agglutinate turkey red blood cells more efficiently than chicken red blood cells. This
results in HA titers of stock CIV approximately fourfold higher and HI titers
for CIV antibodies also fourfold higher on average (E.J. Dubovi, unpublished
observations). With standard serologic tests, antibody responses to CIV can be
detected as early as 8 to 10 days after infection (6–8 days after the onset of clinical signs). This detectable serologic response time coincides with the loss of
virus isolation capability within the same period.

As a word of caution, practitioners should not develop tunnel vision when
dealing with respiratory infections. Although CIV is the emphasis of this article, sampling of sick animals should be done to achieve a diagnosis regardless
of the pathogen. Parallel samples should be collected for detecting bacteria and
mycoplasma in the event that a viral agent is not present. Samples for PCR and
VI should not be collected and put into bacterial transport media. Contact your
diagnostic laboratory for proper sample submission.

MANAGEMENT AND CONTROL

At the present time, there are no licensed vaccines for CIV because there is
some debate as to the significance of CIV as a canine pathogen. For those in
the high-risk areas, the question arose as to the possible use of the equine vaccines, given the close genetic relation between the equine viruses and CIV. Initial immunization with a killed equine vaccine based on an older equine isolate
did not show promising results. Immunization of dogs with a canary poxvirus–
vectored vaccine expressing the HA gene of equine/Ohio/03 or equine /KT/94
produced substantial antibody titers as measured by HI and Nt using canine/
NY/05 as a reference antigen, however [15]. Although no challenge studies
were done, the magnitude of the antibody titers strongly suggested that protective titers to CIV had developed. A limited challenge trial was done using dogs
that had been immunized with a novel equine herpesvirus-vectored vaccine
expressing the HA gene of equine/Ohio/03 [14]. Vaccinated dogs challenged
with canine/PA/07 showed reduced clinical signs and virus shedding as compared with unvaccinated controls. These data show that immunization with
just the HA gene, even from a mismatched equine isolate, was capable of providing some protection to dogs challenged with CIV.

The rather slow spread of CIV in the canine population, as evidenced by the
currently limited geographic distribution of the virus, could provide an opportunity to eradicate CIV. A targeted vaccination program aimed at shelters,
boarding kennels, and racetracks in the affected regions could reduce the level
of infection to a point at which the virus is no longer circulating. This approach
was used in Australia to stem the outbreak of equine influenza virus in 2007.
Restriction of dog movement could not be used, as was done with horses,
but the "contagiousness" of CIV seems to be much less than its counterpart
in horses. Stopping the spread of CIV in dogs before it evolves into a more virulent virus should be the goal of animal disease control officials.

SUMMARY

Based on current information, CIV is an H3N8 type A influenza virus of equine origin that first began causing disease in racing greyhounds in Florida in the early part of the twenty-first century. In most cases, the disease is associated with rescued, kenneled, or boarded dogs characterized by a low-grade fever, persistent cough, and eventual nasal discharge. Attack rates are high, distinguishing CIV infections from other causes of kennel cough. Thankfully, mortality rates are generally low. Rarely, and only reported in racing greyhounds, a severe, often fatal, hemorrhagic pneumonia may develop that may or may not be associated with concurrent streptococcal infections. Nasal swabs seem to be the best sample for confirming a diagnosis. Although licensed vaccines are currently unavailable, they are under development and may be the best means possible for preventing further outbreaks.

References

[1] Nikitin T, Cohen D, Todd JD, et al. Epidemiological studies of A/Hong Kong/68 virus infection in dogs. Bull World Health Organ 1972;47:471–9.

[2] Kilbourne ED, Kehoe JM. Demonstration of antibodies to both hemagglutinin and neuraminidase antigens of H3H2 influenza A virus in domestic dogs. Intervirology 1975/76;6:315–8.

[3] Songserm T, Amonsin A, Jam-on R, et al. Fatal avian influenza A H5N1 in a dog. Emerg Infect Dis 2006;12:1744–6.

[4] Amonsin A, Songserm T, Chutinimitkul S, et al. Genetic analysis of influenza A virus (H5N1) derived from domestic cat and dog in Thailand. Arch Virol 2007;152:1925–33.

[5] Maas R, Tacken M, Ruuls L, et al. Avian influenza (H5N1) susceptibility and receptors in dogs. Emerg Infect Dis 2007;13:1219–21.

[6] Zini E, Glaus TM, Bussadori C, et al. Evaluation of the presence of selected viral and bacterial nucleic acids in pericardial samples from dogs with or without idiopathic pericardial effusion. Vet J 2007, in press.

[7] Giese M, Harder TC, Teifke JP, et al. Experimental infection and natural contact exposure of dogs with avian influenza virus (H5N1). Emerg Infect Dis 2008;14:308–10.

[8] Crawford PC, Dubovi EJ, Castleman WL, et al. Transmission of equine influenza virus to dogs. Science 2005;310:482–5.

[9] Yoon K-J, Cooper VL, Schwartz KJ, et al. Influenza virus infection in racing greyhounds. Emerg Infect Dis 2005;11:1974–5.

[10] Payungporn S, Crawford PC, Kouo, TS, et al. Isolation and characterization of influenza A subtype H3N8 viruses from dogs with respiratory disease in Florida. Emerg Infect Dis 2008, in press.

[11] Available at: http://diagcenter.vet.cornell.edu. Accessed 2005.

[12] Daly JM, Blunden AS, MacRae S, et al. Transmission of equine influenza virus to English foxhounds. Emerg Infect Dis 2008;14:461–4.

[13] Newton R, Cooke A, Elton D, et al. Canine influenza virus: cross-species transmission from horses. Vet Rec 2007;161:142–3.

[14] Rosas C, Van de Walle GR, Metzger SM, et al. Evaluation of a vectored equine herpesvirus type 1 (EHV-1) vaccine expressing the H3 haemagglutinin in the protection of dogs against canine influenza. Vaccine 2008, in press.

[15] Karaca K, Dubovi EJ, Siger L, et al. Evaluation of the ability of canarypox-vectored equine influenza virus vaccines to induce humoral immune responses against canine influenza viruses in dogs. Am J Vet Res 2007;68:208–12.

Vet Clin Small Anim 38 (2008) 837–850

VETERINARY CLINICS
SMALL ANIMAL PRACTICE

Parvovirus Infection in Domestic Companion Animals

Catherine G. Lamm, DVM*, Grant B. Rezabek, MPH, DVM

Oklahoma Animal Disease Diagnostic Laboratory, Oklahoma State University,
Center for Veterinary Health Sciences, PO Box 7001, Stillwater, OK 74076-7001, USA

Parvoviruses are nonenveloped single-stranded DNA viruses that are known to cause disease in a variety of mammalian species. Most parvoviruses are species-specific and infect organs with rapidly dividing cells, such as the intestine, bone marrow, and lymphoid tissue [1].

Parvovirus infection in cats has been known for more than 100 years and is now commonly referred to as feline panleukopenia (FPV) [2]. In 1967, parvovirus was first discovered as a cause of gastrointestinal and respiratory disease in dogs and was coined minute virus of canines [3]. Later, this strain of canine parvovirus (CPV) was designated CPV 1, after the emergence of the antigenically and genomically distinct CPV 2 (Fig. 1). The emergence of CPV 2 in dogs was first reported by several researchers during 1978 to 1982 [4]. CPV 2 caused severe enteritis and high mortality in canine populations.

Over time, the evolution of FPV and CPV 1 has remained relatively stable. This is in strong contrast to CPV 2, which has evolved quickly over the 30-year period since its discovery [5]. Furthermore, mutations in CPV 2 have allowed the virus to spread from the dog to other species, such as the domestic cat and other wild carnivores [6]. This article briefly discusses these three diseases, with emphasis on virus evolution and the challenges to protecting susceptible companion animal populations.

VIRUS STRUCTURE

Parvovirus is spherical and lacks an envelope, and the genome consists of approximately 5000 bases of single-stranded DNA with hair pins at the ends. Like all nonenveloped viruses, parvoviruses are extremely resistant to chemical and environmental inactivation. The virus capsid contains viral protein-1 (VP-1) and VP-2, which allow the virus to bind the host cell transferrin receptor. Interestingly, host susceptibility for CPV and FPV depends on this capsid protein and its ability to bind the host receptor [1,7,8]. Adaptation of this capsid protein to the receptors of other hosts allows efficient transspecies spread, as

*Corresponding author. E-mail address: cathy.lamm@okstate.edu (C.G. Lamm).

0195-5616/08/$ – see front matter
doi:10.1016/j.cvsm.2008.03.008

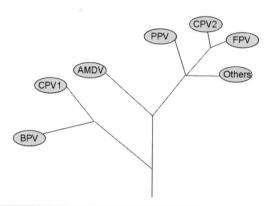

Fig. 1. Evolutionary tree of parvovirus in domestic animals. CPV 1 is closely related to BPV. CPV 2 and FPV are closely related, and both are distinct from CPV 1. AMDV, Aleutian mink disease virus; BPV, bovine parvovirus; PPV, porcine parvovirus. (*Modified from* Ohshima T, Kishi M, Mochizuki M. Sequence analysis of an Asian isolate of minute virus of canines (canine parvovirus type 1). Virus Genes 2004;29(3):294; with permission.)

seen in the spread for the newer strains of CPV 2 from dogs to cats [1]. The capsid protein structure consists of threefold spikes and peaks, which are the major antigenic sites for neutralizing antibodies [1]. FPV penetration and replication within the host cell can occur in the presence of neutralizing antibodies, however [9].

Parvovirus requires the host cell for replication, binding the host cell by the double-stranded ends of the genome. Because of this, parvovirus often infects rapidly dividing cells, including intestinal crypt epithelial cells [10]. Parvovirus' tropism for rapidly dividing cells, such as the enterocytes, leads to clinical disease and death [10]. Viral infection and cytokine-mediated cell death of rapidly dividing cells drive infection and are significant contributors to the development of clinical disease [11].

CANINE PARVOVIRUS 1 (MINUTE VIRUS OF CANINES)
Origin and Virus Strains
CPV 1, or minute virus of canines, is an autonomous virus of unknown origin [3]. CPV 1 is most closely related to bovine parvovirus, with 43% DNA identity [12,13]. CPV 1 is distinct from CPV 2 [13]. The DNA sequence of CPV 1 has remained relatively stable over the past 30 years with greater than 92% homology among CPV 1 strains worldwide [13].

Clinical Signs and Antemortem Testing
Infection of CPV 1 can occur oronasally or transplacentally [14]. After infection, viral replication occurs within lymphatic tissues and intestinal epithelium [15]. Most infections are asymptomatic, and most infected animals do not show clinical signs [15]. Clinical signs vary from sudden death to vomiting, diarrhea, and dyspnea. CPV 1 infection can lead to mortality in pups less than 4 weeks

of age and to reproductive failure in pregnant bitches [14]. Serum neutralizing antibodies against CPV 1 can be detected within 7 days of infection. Virus can also be detected in lymphatic tissue and feces with fluorescent antibody (FA) and electron microscopy [15].

Gross and Histologic Pathologic Findings

The gross changes within affected animals are typically minimal. When present, the intestinal contents are typically liquid and pale streaks may be seen within the heart [14]. In experimental infections, multifocal areas of pulmonary consolidation have been noted [16].

Histologically, there is individual cell necrosis within the intestinal crypts, with crypt hyperplasia and intranuclear inclusion bodies [14]. There is extensive necrosis within the lymphoid tissues, including the Peyer's patches and thymus [15]. Myocardial necrosis and interstitial pneumonia are frequently observed [14,16,17]. Intranuclear inclusion bodies are frequently present within affected organs, particularly within the epithelial cells, such as within the crypt epithelial cells and bronchiolar lining epithelial cells [16].

Infection with CPV 1 can be confirmed on postmortem examination with characteristic histopathologic findings and virus isolation on fresh tissues [16]. FA testing has also been used historically in the diagnosis of CPV 1 infection, although it is not widely performed, because most current commercial FA conjugates offered do not cross-react with CPV 1.

Treatment and Prevention

There is little published information regarding treatment of CPV 1; however, supportive care, including fluids, should be considered on initial presentation of suspected cases. There is also little information available regarding prevention of CPV 1, and the efficacy of current CPV 2 vaccines against CPV 1 challenge is not known.

CANINE PARVOVIRUS 2

Origin and Virus Strains

The origin of CPV has been a topic of great debate. Some speculate that CPV 2 has originated from FPV. Others have shown that the three to four nucleotide differences between FPV and CPV 2 suggest that CPV 2 originated from an antigenically similar ancestor, such as a wild carnivore [6,18–20]. To date, the exact evolution and origin of CPV 2 remain elusive.

Initially, the emergence of CPV 2 in the naive animal population resulted in high morbidity and high mortality. After introduction of vaccines into the canine population, outbreaks were limited to unvaccinated or improperly vaccinated animals and shelter situations with feral or abandoned populations. In the 1980s, a new CPV 2 strain emerged and was designated CPV 2a [21]. Initially, vaccines for CPV 2 seemed to be effective for both strains of the virus. The virus quickly mutated again, and a new strain, CPV 2b, emerged [21]. Recently, vaccine failures occurred in animals infected with CPV 2b, suggesting that the vaccine offered only partial protection in these cases [22].

Within the past few years, a new strain, CPV 2c, has emerged. This strain was first reported in Europe [23] and was soon reported in the United States [24–26]. This strain is highly virulent, often devastating canine populations, with high morbidity and rapid death. Furthermore, as discussed elsewhere in this article, there is significant debate within the scientific community about the efficacy of the current vaccines against CPV 2c.

CPV 2 has tremendous capacity to evolve. Single base changes often translate to dramatic phenotypic changes [27]. These phenotypic changes have resulted in changes in host range and altered immune responses within affected animals [27]. The Glu-426 mutant of CPV 2c has emerged as an important variant and has become the predominant variant over the past 10 years [27]. This mutation affects the major antigenic determinant: the threefold spike of the capsid.

Clinical Signs, Clinical Pathologic Findings, and Antemortem Testing

On exposure of naive animals to the feces of CPV 2–infected animals or fomites having contacted infected animals, viral replication occurs within the oropharynx. Virus is disseminated through the blood to a variety of organs, resulting in systemic infection [28]. The primary pathologic site for viral replication is within the intestinal crypts, resulting in profound enteritis and diarrhea [29]. The incubation period is 3 days to 1 week between initial infection and the onset of clinical signs [19].

Parvovirus does not affect all dogs equally, with different strains resulting in varied effects based on the age of the animal, immunity, breed, route of exposure, viral dose, and virulence of the strain [29]. Typically, parvovirus infection peaks after weaning at the age of 4 to 12 weeks, when maternal antibodies wane. Infection can be seen commonly in pups up to 6 months of age, however [19]. Clinical signs in some puppies may be unapparent. The most common clinical signs include vomiting and diarrhea. The diarrhea can range from mucoid to bloody. Dehydration and secondary infection often develop rapidly. Clinically, animals often have severe, although transient, leukopenia with counts as low as 500 to 2000 white blood cells (WBCs)/μL [10,19,29,30]. Lymphopenia is often more pronounced than neutropenia. Anemia can be present but is not a consistent feature of infection [10]. Death can occur as quickly as 24 hours after the onset of clinical signs, especially in younger animals [29]. Infection associated with clinical disease is rare in adult dogs but has been recently been observed with CPV 2c outbreaks in the United States [19].

Antemortem diagnosis is confirmed by clinical signs, history, and elimination of other causes of diarrhea [29]. Commercial tests are available for patient-side use [31]. Such tests detect antigen in fecal material and have relatively high specificity but low sensitivity [32]. Inappropriate vaccination methods (ie, oral) can result in false-positive results. Modified-live vaccines can also yield false-positive results in dogs 4 to10 days after vaccination, when administered appropriately [19].

During a 1-year period, more than 50% of cases that were confirmed as parvovirus at necropsy at the Oklahoma Animal Disease Diagnostic Laboratory were SNAP test-negative before death (C.G. Lamm and G.B. Rezabek, personal observation, 2006). This finding is similar to that of another recently published study, which found that the SNAP test was only able to detect 46% of infected dogs [32]. The cause of the SNAP test failure could be related to decreased viral shedding, because virus is only detectable in feces 10 to 12 days after infection [19]. Improper test procedure can also affect the outcome of the test. Interestingly, the increase in SNAP test failure has paralleled the emergence of CPV 2c. This circumstantial evidence is suggestive that the current test used has a low cross-reactivity for the new strain of virus (CPV 2c).

Gross and Histologic Pathologic Findings

Parvoviruses cause a wide range of gross and histologic changes that vary from minimal to severe. At necropsy, the most common finding is segmental enteritis (Fig. 2). The serosa of the affected areas is often dark red, rough, and pitted, and the mucosa is often smooth and glassy because of loss of villi. The small intestinal contents can vary from watery to yellow mucoid or bloody or hemorrhagic. On occasion, minimal lesions are noted on gross examination [33].

Sample selection for histology is critical, with segments of bowel being variably affected. The virus typically infects the proximal small intestine first and progresses segmentally down the small intestine. The large intestine is rarely affected. In the acute cases, there is multifocal crypt necrosis and intranuclear inclusion bodies are frequently observed in the intestine. As the disease progresses, there is loss of crypt architecture with villus blunting, fusion, or sloughing, and crypt regeneration (Fig. 3). In chronic cases, inclusions are rare, which correlates with decreased CPV 2 antigen detection [33]. Secondary bacterial infection is a common finding and can be a significant cofactor for mortality in less virulent parvovirus cases. Multiple noncontinuous segments of small intestine should be harvested for confirmation.

Although the small intestine has the most striking histologic changes, viral inclusions can be appreciated in a variety of organ systems, particularly the

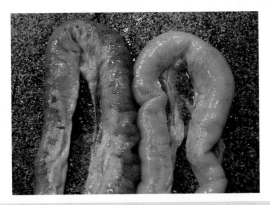

Fig. 2. Intestine from a dog with acute parvovirus infection. There is segmental enteritis, with the affected segment on the left and the unaffected segment on the right.

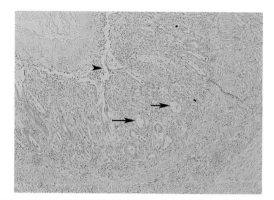

Fig. 3. Photomicrograph of the intestine from a dog with parvovirus infection. There is marked crypt necrosis (*arrows*) with villus blunting (*arrowhead*).

heart. Myocarditis with intranuclear inclusion bodies can be seen in a fraction of cases, especially in younger animals (Fig. 4) [33]. Depletion of the erythroid and myeloid lines and of the megakaryocytes within the bone marrow is also seen [9].

In early stages, immunohistochemistry can be used on sections of intestine and tongue to confirm infection [34]. In later stages, because of loss of detectable antigen, the immunohistochemical stain may be falsely negative. Other tests, such as hemagglutination testing, FA testing, virus isolation, and polymerase chain reaction (PCR), are available at diagnostic laboratories. Hemagglutination inhibition detects antigen within fecal homogenate. Virus isolation and PCR can be performed on feces or sections of fresh intestine or tongue. FA testing can be performed on sections of fresh intestine and tongue. Of these tests, PCR is the most accurate, detecting more than 90% of infected animals [32].

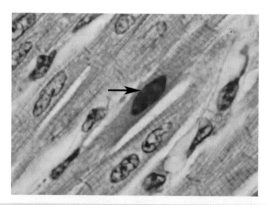

Fig. 4. Photomicrograph of the heart from a dog with parvovirus infection. There are distinct intranuclear inclusion bodies (*arrow*). (*Courtesy of* Gregory A. Campbell, DVM, PhD, Stillwater, OK.)

Genotyping of the PCR product is available at most full-service diagnostic laboratories.

Treatment and Prevention

The treatment of parvovirus infection in individual animals is supportive and symptom based. Management of dehydration with fluids is critical. Transfusions may be necessary in severe cases. Prevention of secondary intestinal bacterial infection is also important, and administration of antibiotics is recommended. Antiemetics to manage severe vomiting and corticosteroids to treat endotoxic shock may be needed and can be used symptomatically. In severe cases, restriction of oral intake of food and water may be necessary. Antidiarrheal medications are contraindicated. With appropriate care, most parvovirus cases (75%) should respond to medical therapy [35]. Recovered animals maintain protective immunity against that strain for life [29].

Parvovirus is highly contagious and can be devastating in kennel and shelter situations. Viral shedding can occur up to 2 weeks or longer, and affected animals should be isolated during this period [30]. Precautions should be taken to prevent spread by means of fomites between areas with affected and unaffected animals. Parvovirus is highly resistant to inactivation and can persist in the environment for months to years [30]. Housing, bedding, and other material in contact with affected animals should be thoroughly cleaned with a dilute bleach solution on a regular basis.

There are several effective brands of CPV 2 vaccines on the market depending on the strain of parvovirus circulating within the population. Vaccination of dogs is recommended. The susceptibility window for infection with CPV in pups with adequate maternal antibodies actually begins 2 to 3 weeks before the waning of maternal antibodies at 8 to 12 weeks of age. Given the presence of maternal antibodies, vaccination ranges in effectiveness from 25% in 6-week-old pups to 95% in 18-week-old pups. To maximize the effectiveness of vaccination, a series of vaccinations over this window is recommended. The vaccination schedule should be developed on a case-by-case basis with consideration of age, environment, and the recommendations of the package insert literature for the vaccine being used. In general, core vaccination of a modified-live vaccine at 6 to 8 weeks, 9 to 11 weeks, and 12 to 16 weeks of age is recommended. A booster vaccination should be administered 1 year later and then every 1 to 3 years [29,36]. Parvovirus-related disease can occur after vaccination. It has been shown that most of these cases are related to infection with a wild-type strain and not reversion of the modified-live vaccine strain [37]. Infection with variant strains, overwhelming viral dose, and route of exposure are additional factors that can be responsible for clinical illness in vaccinated animals.

Evolution of Canine Parvovirus 2 and Today's Challenges

Up until the past 5 to 6 years, CPV infection has remained a relatively treatable and preventable disease. Severe mortality rates were often reserved for shelter outbreak situations in groups of naive, unvaccinated, stressed animals.

Recently, parvovirus has become an issue within well-managed and well-vaccinated animals, especially in breeding situations. Furthermore, in a disease that is usually mainly restricted to younger animals, adult vaccinated animals are also developing diarrhea with rare mortality.

The cause for this shift in clinical presentation and mortality rates is manyfold. The CPV virus has rapidly evolved over the past 30 years, and there are now four separate types circulating within different countries [23,38,39]. With each evolutionary shift, there is altered protection from maternal antibodies and vaccination [5,20]. Recently, the emergence of CPV 2c is the most challenging. Not only does the detection of CPV 2c seem to be limited with modern antigen detection kits, but current vaccines seem to have questionable protection [24]. Furthermore, the US canine population remains relatively naive to this new strain, lacking any circulating antibodies. These factors are ideal for outbreak situations with high morbidity and high mortality. The CPV 2 vaccine seems to confer a lower level of immunity of shorter duration against the CPV 2b biotype than against the original strain [40].

The presence of the CPV 2c variant has also raised questions about the efficacy of the current vaccines against this new strain. Some researchers report that some vaccines on the market protect against European strains of CPV 2c [41–43]. Other researchers have reported limited serum neutralization capabilities of vaccinated animals against European CPV 2c strains [44,45]. Furthermore, some researchers have shown that the older CPV 2 vaccines do not offer protection against CPV 2c [22]. The efficacy of current vaccines against CPV 2c strains circulating within the United States has yet to be determined.

In addition to antigenic drift, secondary bacterial infections are playing an increasing role in the high mortality rates associated with parvovirus infection. Bacterial infections are often related to overgrowth and invasion of commensal organisms and secondary invaders, such as *Salmonella*, β-hemolytic *Escherichia coli*, and *Clostridium difficile*. Furthermore, antibiotic-resistant strains are more prevalent and possibly overrepresented in large and intensively managed breeding facilities. Overgrowth and invasion of these organisms can result in systemic release of toxins or systemic infection. These secondary infections pose a new challenge for practitioners in the treatment of CPV 2–infected animals.

Canine Parvovirus 2 Infection in Cats

The original strain of CPV 2 is not associated with disease in cats [1]. CPV 2a and CPV 2b have been shown to infect cats, however, causing severe enteritis [6,46]. It is interesting to note that these later strains contain a mutation around the capsid protein encoded by the VP-2 residue 300 [1,47]. In cats, CPV 2a or 2b infection results in clinical presentation, progression, and mortality rates similar to those in dogs. Furthermore, infection with CPV 2a or 2b in cats can be difficult to distinguish from infection with FPV. In cats, vaccination with the FPV vaccine has been shown to be protective against infection with CPV 2a and CPV 2b [48].

FELINE PANLEUKOPENIA
Origin and Host Range
FPV was first described more than 100 years ago. The origin of the virus remains unknown, and the evolution of the virus has remained relatively stable, with little variation in the virus genome over time [2]. In addition to causing significant disease in domestic cats, FPV is able to infect a wide variety of wild felids and other wild carnivores [49]. FPV does not readily replicate within domestic canids and is not associated with clinical disease in this species [1].

Clinical Signs, Clinical Pathologic Findings, and Antemortem Testing
FPV is spread by means of direct contact with the secretions of virus-infected cats, including feces, urine, and blood, and can also be transmitted transplacentally. Fleas have been shown to be a vector for FPV [50]. Infection in adults and kittens is characterized by fever, vomiting, and diarrhea. In utero infections with FPV can result in abortion, mummified fetuses, and stillbirth.

After exposure of kittens and adults to the virus, FPV first infects the oropharynx, followed by rapid viremia. The incubation period before the onset of clinical signs is 4 to 5 days, and the clinical course can rapidly progress to death [50]. The primary pathologic site for viral replication is within the intestinal crypts because of the high mitotic activity, resulting in profound enteritis and diarrhea. Lymphoid tissue is also a target, resulting in profound pancytopenia with cell counts less than 4000 cells/µL [50]. Thrombocytopenia may also be seen. In the later stages of disease, a rebounding increase in WBC counts can be seen. A nonregenerative anemia can also be seen in recovering patients [50]. Icterus accompanied by an increase in bilirubin may also be noted in some cases.

Clinical signs, serology for FPV antibodies, and fecal tests for FPV antigen are useful methods for the diagnosis of FPV infection [50]. Recent vaccination can give false-positive results [51].

Gross and Histologic Pathologic Findings
With infection in kittens and adult cats, the most common finding at postmortem examination is segmental enteritis, similar to that in CPV infection. As with CPV 2, the histologic changes within the small intestine include multifocal crypt necrosis, loss of crypt architecture with villus blunting, and crypt regeneration (Fig. 5). In chronic cases, inclusions are rare, which correlates with decreased antigen detection [33]. Secondary bacterial infection is a common finding.

With in utero infections, FPV has a teratogenic effect that has a varied result depending on the stage of infection. In the latter stages of gestation, the virus targets the brain and the eye because of the high degree of proliferative activity [50]. This results in cerebellar hypoplasia, hydrocephalus, hydranencephaly, and retinal dysplasia [33].

Immunohistochemistry can be used on sections of intestine and tongue to confirm infection, although false-negative results can occur [34]. FA detection, conventional PCR, and virus isolation may also be used to detect antigen within sections of fresh intestine and tongue. These tests have similar

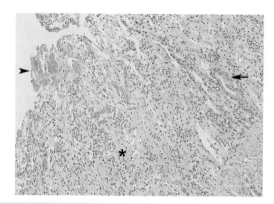

Fig. 5. Photomicrograph of the intestine from a cat with FPV. The histologic changes resemble those in CPV infection with crypt loss (*asterisk*) and regeneration (*arrow*). Abundant bacteria are adherent to the surface (*arrowhead*).

limitations as immunohistochemistry, though PCR is slightly more sensitive. Unfortunately, none of these tests differentiate CPV infection from FPV infection. Recently, a real-time PCR was developed against a single nucleotide difference at the 3753 position (residue 232 of the capsid protein), which differentiates CPV infection from FPV infection [52].

Treatment and Prevention

As with CPV infection, the treatment of parvovirus infection in cats is supportive. Management of dehydration and prevention of secondary intestinal bacterial infection are critical. The withholding of food and water may be necessary until the vomiting is controlled. Administration of antiserum to colostrum-deprived kittens may be useful in the control of outbreaks in group situations [50].

Because parvovirus is nonenveloped, it is highly resistant to disinfection and highly contagious. Affected animals should be isolated, and precautions should be taken to prevent spread by means of fomites between areas with affected and unaffected animals. Housing, bedding, and other material in contact with affected animals should be thoroughly cleaned with a dilute bleach solution. Virus shedding persists up to 6 weeks after cessation of clinical signs. Because of this, recovered animals should remain in isolation for an extended period to prevent transmission [50]. In cattery situations, administration of recombinant feline interferon to the queen before kittling or to kittens before exposure to contaminated areas has been shown to stimulate antibody response and improve survival rates [53].

Vaccination of healthy cats is recommended. There are currently several FPV vaccines on the market that have been shown to have excellent efficacy if administered appropriately. A vaccination schedule should be created on an individual basis with consideration of age, environment, and the recommendations of the package insert literature for the vaccine being used. In general, a core vaccination of a modified-live vaccine at 6 to 8 weeks, 9 to 11 weeks, and 12 to 16 weeks of age is recommended. A booster vaccination should be administered 1 year later and then every 1 to 3 years, depending on risk for exposure [50]. Booster vaccinations every 3 years has been shown to be effective in general feline populations [36,54].

Caution should be used when vaccinating immunocompromised cats, such as those on corticosteroids or those infected with feline immunodeficiency virus. Vaccination of cats that are infected with retroviruses (feline leukemia virus or feline immunodeficiency virus) using the current modified-live FPV vaccines can result in FPV-like disease [55].

Evolution of Feline Panleukopenia

Historically, there has been minimal change in the genome of FPV. A recent study indicated no changes within the amino acid sequence of the VP2 gene, indicating the lack of emergence of new variants [56].

SUMMARY

Parvovirus infects a wide variety of species. The rapid evolution, environmental resistance, high dose of viral shedding, and interspecies transmission have made some strains of parvovirus infection difficult to control within domestic animal populations. Some parvoviruses in companion animals, such as CPV 1 and FPV, have demonstrated minimal evolution over time. A combination of vaccination, sanitation, and limitation of viral burden in kennel situations have helped to control these diseases within the domestic animal populations.

In contrast, CPV 2 has shown wide adaptability with rapid evolution and frequent mutations. These new strains have not only been able to gain a foothold in populations considered to be immune but have shown remarkable capacity to be transmitted between species. Although vaccination has proved to control the spread of CPV to some degree, the rapid mutation of the virus has led to some concern about the efficacy of older vaccines in a domestic canine population that is immunologically naive to the newer strains.

References

[1] Hueffer K, Parrish CR. Parvovirus host range, cell tropism, and evolution. Curr Opin Microbiol 2003;6:392–8.
[2] Squires RA. An update on aspects of viral gastrointestinal diseases of dogs and cats. N Z Vet J 2003;51(6):252–61.
[3] Binn LN, Lazar C, Eddy GA, et al. Recovery and characterization of a minute virus of canines. Infect Immun 1970;1(5):503–8.
[4] Eugster AK, Bendele RA, Jones LP. Parvovirus infection in dogs. J Am Vet Med Assoc 1978;173(10):1340–1.
[5] Truyen U. Evolution of canine parvovirus—a new need for vaccines? Vet Microbiol 2006;117:9–13.
[6] Gamoh K, Shimazaki Y, Makie H, et al. The pathogenicity of canine parvovirus type-2b, FP84 strain isolated from a domestic cat, in domestic cats. J Vet Med Sci 2003;65(9): 1027–9.
[7] Cotmore SF, Tattersall P. Parvoviral host range and cell entry mechanisms. Adv Virus Res 2007;70:183–232.

[8] Govindasamy L, Hueffer K, Parrish CR, et al. Structures of host-range controlling regions of the capsids of canine and feline parvoviruses and mutants. J Virol 2003;77(22):12211–21.

[9] Nelson CD, Palermo LM, Hafenstein SL, et al. Different mechanisms of antibody-mediated neutralization of parvoviruses revealed using the Fab fragments of monoclonal antibodies. Virology 2007;361(2):283–93.

[10] Parrish CR. Pathogenesis of feline panleukopenia virus and canine parvovirus. Baillieres Clin Haematol 1995;8(1):57–71.

[11] Bauder B, Suchy A, Gabler C, et al. Apoptosis in feline panleukopenia and canine parvovirus enteritis. J Vet Med B Infect Dis Vet Public Health 2000;47(10):775–84.

[12] Schwartz D, Green B, Carmicheal LE, et al. The canine minute virus (minute virus of canines) is a distinct parvovirus that is most similar to bovine parvovirus. Virology 2002;302(2): 219–23.

[13] Ohshima T, Kishi M, Mochizuki M. Sequence analysis of an Asian isolate of minute virus of canines (canine parvovirus type 1). Virus Genes 2004;29(3):291–6.

[14] Harrison LR, Styer EL, Pursell AR, et al. Fatal disease in nursing puppies associated with minute virus of canines. J Vet Diagn Invest 1992;4:19–22.

[15] Macartney L, Parrish CR, Binn LN, et al. Characterization of minute virus of canines (MVC) and its pathogenicity for pups. Cornell Vet 1988;78:131–45.

[16] Carmichael LE, Schlafer DH, Hasimoto A. Minute virus of canines (MVC, canine parvovirus type-1): pathogenicity for pups and seroprevalence estimate. J Vet Dlagn Invest 1994;6: 165–74.

[17] Jarplid B, Johansson H, Carmichael LE. A fatal case of pup infection with minute virus of canines. J Vet Diagn Invest 1996;8:484–7.

[18] Carmichael LE. An annotated historical account of canine parvovirus. J Vet Med B Infect Dis Vet Public Health 2005;52:303–11.

[19] Pollock RVH, Coyne MJ. Canine parvovirus. Vet Clin North Am Small Anim Pract 1993;23(3):555–69.

[20] Truyen U. Emergence and recent evolution of canine parvovirus. Vet Microbiol 1999;69: 47–50.

[21] Parrish CR, Have P, Foreyt WJ, et al. The global spread and replacement of canine parvovirus strains. J Gen Virol 1988;69:1111–6.

[22] Desario C, Lorusso E, Nardi M, et al. Outbreak of canine type 2c natural infection in adult dogs repeatedly administered a type 2-based vaccine [abstract P 03]. In: Proceedings of the international parvovirus meeting. Bari (Italy): 2007.

[23] Decaro N, Martella V, Desario C, et al. First detection of canine parvovirus type 2c in pups with haemorrhagic enteritis in Spain. J Vet Med B Infect Dis Vet Public Health 2006;53: 468–72.

[24] Kapil S, Cooper E, Lamm C, et al. Canine parvovirus types 2c and 2b circulating in North American dogs: 2006–2007. J Clin Microbiol 2007;45:4044–7.

[25] Kapil S, Cooper E, Murray B, et al. Canine parvovirus variants circulating in the USA:2006–2007 [abstract OC 01]. In: Proceedings of the international parvovirus meeting. Bari (Italy): 2007.

[26] Hong C, Decaro N, Desario C, et al. Occurrence of canine parvovirus type 2c in the United States. J Vet Diagn Invest 2007;19(5):535–9.

[27] Martella V, Decaro N, Elia G, et al. Surveillance activity for canine parvovirus in Italy. J Vet Med B Infect Dis Vet Public Health 2005;52:312–5.

[28] Meunier PC, Cooper BJ, Appel MJG, et al. Pathogenesis of canine enteritis: sequential virus distribution and passive immunization studies. Vet Pathol 1985;22:617–24.

[29] Sherding RG. Small bowel disease. In: Ettinger SJ, editor. 3rd edition, Textbook of veterinary medicine, vol. 2. Philadelphia: WB Saunders; 1989. p. 1351–3.

[30] Swango LJ. Canine viral diseases. In: Ettinger SJ, editor. Textbook of veterinary medicine, vol. 1. 3rd edition. Philadelphia: WB Saunders; 1989. p. 307–309.

[31] Lacheretz A, Laperrousaz C, Kodjo A, et al. Diagnosis of canine parvovirus by rapid immunomigration on a membrane. Vet Rec 2003;152(2):48–50.
[32] Desario C, Decaro N, Campolo M, et al. Canine parvovirus infection: which diagnostic test for virus? J Virol Methods 2005;126:179–85.
[33] Brown CC, Baker DC, Barker IK. Alimentary system. In: Maxie MG, editor. Pathology of domestic animals, vol. 2. 5th edition. London: Elsevier Saunders; 2007. p. 177–182.
[34] McKnight CA, Maes RK, Wise AG, et al. Evaluation of tongue as a complementary sample for the diagnosis of parvoviral infection in dogs and cats. J Vet Diagn Invest 2007;19: 409–13.
[35] Available at: www.AVMA.org. Accessed November, 2007.
[36] Schultz RD. Duration of immunity for canine and feline vaccines: a review. Vet Microbiol 2006;117:75–9.
[37] Decaro N, Desario C, Elia G, et al. Occurrence of severe gastroenteritis in pups after canine parvovirus vaccine administration: a clinical and laboratory diagnostic dilemma. Vaccine 2007;25(7):1161–6.
[38] Palmer J, Thornley M. Canine parvovirus outbreaks. Aust Vet J 2004;82(12):720.
[39] Shackelton LA, Parrish CR, Truyen U, et al. High rate of viral evolution associated with the emergence of carnivore parvovirus. Proc Natl Acad Sci U S A 2005;102(2):379–84.
[40] Pratelli A, Cavalli A, Martella V, et al. Canine parvovirus (CPV) vaccination: comparison of neutralizing antibody responses in pups after inoculation with CPV2 or CPV2b modified live virus vaccine. Clin Diagn Lab Immunol 2001;8(3):612–5.
[41] Bruent S, Toulemonde C, Cariou C, et al. Efficacy of vaccination with a canine parvovirus type 2 against a virulent challenge with a CPV type 2c (GLU426) [abstract OC 3]. In: Proceedings of the international parvovirus meeting. Bari (Italy): 2007.
[42] Siedek EM, Schmidt H, Munyira P, et al. Vanguard 7 protects against challenge with virulent canine parvovirus antigenic type 2c (CPV 2c) [abstract P 06]. In: Proceedings of the international parvovirus meeting. Bari (Italy): 2007.
[43] Spibey N, Greenwood N, Tarpey I, et al. A canine parvovirus type 2 vaccine protects dogs following challenge with a recent type 2c strain [abstract P 07]. In: Proceedings of the international parvovirus meeting. Bari (Italy): 2007.
[44] Decaro N. Genetic and antigenic evolution of canine parvovirus: global emergence of new variants. A new threat to dogs? [abstract L 02]. In: Proceedings of the international parvovirus meeting. Bari (Italy): 2007.
[45] Cavalli A, Mari V, Moschidou P, et al. Antigenic relationships among canine parvovirus (CPV 2) variants [abstract P 04]. In: Proceedings of the international parvovirus meeting. Bari (Italy): 2007.
[46] Nakamura K, Ikeda Y, Miyazawa T, et al. Characterisation of cross-reactivity of virus neutralising antibodies induced by feline panleukopenia virus and canine parvoviruses. Res Vet Sci 2001;71(3):219–22.
[47] Battilani M, Scagliarini A, Ciulli S, et al. High genetic diversity of the VP 2 gene of a canine parvovirus strain detected in a domestic cat. Virology 2006;352:22–6.
[48] Gamoh K, Senda M, Inoue Y, et al. Efficacy of an inactivated feline panleucopenia virus vaccine against a canine parvovirus isolated from a domestic cat. Vet Rec 2005;157:285–7.
[49] Steinel A, Munsno L, van Vuuren M, et al. Genetic characterization of feline parvovirus sequences from various carnivores. J Gen Virol 2000;81:345–50.
[50] August JR. Feline viral diseases. In: Ettinger SJ, editor. Textbook of veterinary medicine, vol. 1. 3rd edition. Philadelphia: WB Saunders; 1989. p. 314–7.
[51] Patterson EV, Reese MJ, Tucker SJ, et al. Effect of vaccination on parvovirus antigen testing in kittens. J Am Vet Med Assoc 2007;230(3):359–63.
[52] Decaro N, Desario C, Lucente MS, et al. Specific identification of feline panleukopenia virus and its rapid differentiation from canine parvovirus using minor grove binder probes. J Virol Methods 2008;147(1):67–71.

[53] Paltrinieri S, Crippa A, Comerio T, et al. Evaluation of inflammation and immunity in cats with spontaneous parvovirus infection: consequences of recombinant feline interferon administration. Vet Immunol Immunopathol 2007;118(1–2):68–74.

[54] Gore TC, Lakshmanan N, Williams JR, et al. Thee-year duration of immunity in cats following vaccination against feline rhinotracheitis virus, feline calicivirus, and feline panleukopenia virus. Vet Ther 2006;7(3):213–22.

[55] Buonavoglia C, Marsilio F, Tempesta M, et al. Use of a feline panleukopenia modified live virus vaccine in cats in the primary-stage of feline immunodeficiency virus infection. Zentralbl Veterinarmed B 1993;40(5):343–6.

[56] Battilani M, Bassani M, Ustulin M, et al. Molecular evolution of feline parvovirus (FPV) [abstract P 01]. In: Proceedings of the international parvovirus meeting. Bari (Italy).

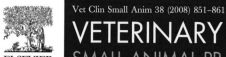
Vet Clin Small Anim 38 (2008) 851–861

VETERINARY CLINICS
SMALL ANIMAL PRACTICE

Rabies in Small Animals

Sarah N. Lackay, MS, Yi Kuang, MD, Zhen F. Fu, DVM, PhD*

Department of Pathology, College of Veterinary Medicine, University of Georgia,
501 D.W. Brooks Drive, CVM Building, Athens, GA 30602-7388, USA

R abies is an ancient disease, and its history can be traced back more than 5000 years [1]. Despite significant scientific progress, rabies remains an important global disease. Annually, more than 55,000 human fatalities are reported, and millions of others require postexposure treatment [2,3]. Most of the human cases occur in the developing nations of Asia and Africa, where dog rabies remains endemic or epizootic, and is thus the main source for human exposure [1]. In developed countries, human rabies has dramatically declined during the past 60 years as a direct consequence of routine vaccination of pet animals.

RABIES IN THE UNITED STATES

In the United States, rabies was once endemic in small animals, particularly in dogs, and thus was a major public health problem in the beginning of the past century. Approximately 10,000 rabies cases were reported annually in dogs and cats [4]. Massive immunizations in domestic dogs and cats were initiated in the 1940s and 1950s. As a consequence, rabies in dogs and cats declined dramatically; now, only a few hundred cases are reported each year (Fig. 1) [4]. The rabies virus strains that used to be associated with dogs have disappeared during the last few years [5]. Viruses associated with small animals are derived from strains affecting wildlife.

Currently wildlife rabies is enzootic in the United States. Seven to eight thousand cases have been reported in wildlife annually during the past 2 decades [5,6]. Concurrently, there are a few rabies enzootics occurring in the United States. The distribution of the terrestrial animal rabies epizootics is shown in Fig. 2 [7]. Raccoon rabies spread along the eastern seaboard during the 1980s and 1990s [8] and has been spreading westward in the new century [9]. Three different variants exist in striped skunks in long-standing reservoirs in California, the north central states, and the south central states [10]. Skunks have now been reported to be infected with raccoon and bat rabies variants in other states [11,12]. There are at least three fox rabies enzootics: Arctic foxes in

*Corresponding author. E-mail address: zhenfu@uga.edu (Z.F. Fu).

0195-5616/08/$ – see front matter
doi:10.1016/j.cvsm.2008.03.003

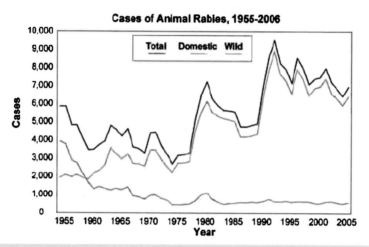

Fig. 1. Cases of animal rabies in the United States, by year, 1955 through 2006. (*From* Blanton JD, Hanlon CA, Rupprecht CE. Rabies surveillance in the United States during 2006. J Am Vet Med Assoc 2007;231:541; with permission.)

Alaska, along with red and gray foxes in the Southeast [13,14]. Some of these terrestrial wildlife species may have acquired rabies virus from dogs a long time ago, which has adapted to these species and their locations since [15]. Other rabies viruses may have evolved from bat rabies variants [12]. Spillover from one species to another occurs from time to time [12,16] and may lead to spreading in the new species. The distribution of these terrestrial rabies epizootics are depicted in Fig. 2A, and the phylogenetic relation of these rabies variants in the United States is summarized in Fig. 2B [7]. In addition to terrestrial animal rabies, bat rabies has been detected in all the 48 contiguous states and has been responsible for most of the human cases in the United States for the past 20 years [5].

Wildlife rabies presents a health problem to domestic small animals, which, in turn, have a higher risk for transmission to human beings because of their close contact with people. Rabies variants found in domestic animals include variants found in raccoons, north central skunks, south central skunks, Texas foxes, Texas dog-coyotes, and California skunks [17].

RABIES IN DOGS

Dogs are the natural host for rabies. There are two forms of rabies—the excitatory or "furious" form and the paralytic or "dumb" form [18,19]. There are several overlapping phases during the progression of the disease: the prodromal period, the furious period, and the paralytic period [18,19]. The clinical signs of rabies may vary among animals, however. The first stage lasts 2 to 3 days in dogs. During this phase, infected animals always show different behavior. The excitement phase may last up to a week, but animals sometimes

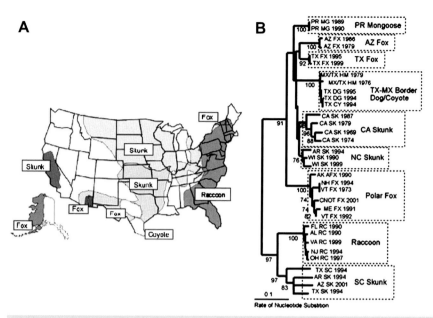

Fig. 2. (A) Geographic distribution of the major terrestrial carnivore hosts of rabies virus variants. Each region is largely characterized by a unique rabies variant specific to a single carnivore host. (B) Neighbor-joining tree for nucleotide sequence of a 320–base pair region of the nucleoprotein gene of selected rabies virus (RABV) isolates from the United States, Mexico, and Canada. Each group of virus isolates that was sequenced to illustrate the unique RABV variants associated with terrestrial carnivores is boxed. The Polar fox variant (Arctic and red fox) is no longer considered enzootic in the United States. Bootstrap values are shown at the branching point for clades recovered in >700/1000 iterations of the data. Australian bat lyssavirus was used as the outgroup and to root the tree. Samples from a rabid fox in Ontario, Canada (CN OT FX 2/4) and from two human rabies cases with exposures to rabid dogs in Mexico (MX/TX HM 1976 and 1979) are included to show variants of RABV shared across international boundaries. US samples are identified by a two-letter abbreviation for the state and animal from which the sample originated, followed by the year the case occurred. With the exception of the Canadian sample (GenBank accession U11735), all RABV sequences were derived from samples in a virus repository at the Centers for Disease Control and Prevention. (*From* Real LA, Russell C, Waller L, et al. Spatial dynamics and molecular ecology of North American rabies. J Hered 2005;96:258; with permission.)

progress directly from the prodromal phase to the paralytic stage. In the second period, animals suddenly become vicious and behave erratically. Within several days, the disease progresses to the paralytic stage. In the last period, animals show paralysis, first in the wounded limb and then in the neck and head. Disease in animals ends in respiratory failure and death [18,19]. The course of rabies typically lasts 3 to 8 days in dogs.

Recently, a report described rabies symptoms in a 6-month-old, mixed-breed, female dog in Florida, which provides valuable insight into clinical presentation of rabies meningoencephalomyelitis. At presentation, the dog had a 3-day history of acute paraplegia, including areflexia, hyperesthesia, and nonpainful swelling of the left second and third digits of the affected limb, eventually progressing to flaccid paralysis of the right pelvic limb. Analysis of lumbar cerebrospinal fluid (CSF) showed abnormally high protein, red blood cell (RBC), and white blood cell (WBC) counts. Cytopathologic examination revealed 78% lymphocytes, 21% mononuclear phagocytes, and 1% neutrophils. Serum testing results for rabies neutralization antibodies using the rapid fluorescent focus inhibition test (RFFIT) were negative. Electromyography (EMG) of left pelvic limb revealed moderate fibrillations and positive sharp waves suggestive of denervation or myopathy. No M wave could be generated for the left sciatic nerve, indicating a lack of axonal or neuromuscular transmission. F waves were also absent on the left sciatic, tibial, and ulnar nerves. Results for the right limb, paravertebral muscles, and thoracic limb muscles and for the right sciatic, tibial, and ulnar nerves were normal. Dementia, salivation, and development of bilateral ventrolateral strabismus, focal and facial limb seizure, and aggression occurred on recovery from anesthesia. After euthanasia, the animal tested positive for raccoon rabies. Intracytoplasmic inclusion bodies could be seen in the brain stem and spinal cord. Degenerate and necrotic neurons were seen within the thoracic and lumbar spinal cord [20].

It is interesting to note that there have been cases of cerebral cysticercosis caused by the larval *Taenia solium*, which mimics rabies virus infection in dogs [21]. Additionally, there have been cases of cutaneous vasculitis associated with rabies vaccine administration in dogs, all with a similar inflammatory pattern of mononuclear cells (nonleukocytoclastic) [22].

RABIES IN CATS

Cats are the domestic animals most frequently reported rabid in the United States, and 200 to 300 cases are reported annually [23]. In one study in Pennsylvania, 44% of human postexposure prophylaxis (PEP) was attributable to exposure to a potentially rabid cat [16]. Factors influencing the increased incidence of rabies in cats include community tolerance of free-ranging felines and less frequent rabies vaccination because of more lenient state laws for cats as compared with dogs. Additionally, communities of feral cats exist, and people who care for these feral animals are at risk for coming into contact with rabies virus. Cats are predominantly affected by the variant of rabies virus endemic to the region in which they reside. For example, along the North American eastern coast, cats are commonly infected with the raccoon rabies virus variant. Cats can also contract bat rabies virus variants, however, because cats and bats are both nocturnal and cats trap small animals like bats [24]. Rabid cats display symptoms similar to those in dogs but have a tendency to hide in secluded places and are often more vicious. Similar to recommendations for dogs, it is a common recommendation to confine and observe a cat involved in a human bite to rule out rabies exposure [24,25].

RABIES IN OTHER SMALL ANIMALS

In addition to dogs and cats, rabies has been reported in other domestic small animals, such as ferrets and rabbits. Two species of ferrets are common in the United States: the common ferret (*Mustela putorius*) and the black-footed ferret (*Mustela nigripes*). Ferrets have become popular companion animals in the United States. Ferrets were originally used to hunt small game and suckling animals and may be attracted by the smell of milk [26]. Although rare, rabid pet ferrets have been reported in the United States [6]. Therefore, it has become increasingly important to be aware of clinical signs of rabies in domestic ferrets to avoid potentially harmful interactions with their human owners. Clinical signs of paralytic rabies in ferrets include lethargy, ataxia, paresis, paraparesis, paralysis, bladder atony, constipation, hypothermia, inappetence and anorexia, abnormal or frequent vocalization, sneezing, paresthesia, and ptyalism (moist or matted fur around the mouth). Only approximately 10% of rabid ferrets in experimental infection showed aggressive behavior with rapid attack and destruction toward a paper applicator; most had no to mild interest in the applicator. It has been recommended to vaccinate all pet ferrets against rabies and to consider rabies in the differential diagnosis of ferrets with acute personality change or paralysis [27,28].

Rabies cases have also been reported in rodents and lagomorphs, including a rabid pet guinea pig in 2003, which bit its owner in the clavicle. The guinea pig was later found to be infected with raccoon rabies virus. Between 1991 and 2001, the Wadsworth Center Rabies Laboratory received seven lagomorphs, all pet domestics, three of which were exposed to a raccoon and one to a skunk. All seven lagomorphs were infected with raccoon rabies virus [29]. Rodents and lagomorphs should be considered "spillover" species rather than reservoirs, however. Unfortunately, clinical signs are often not obvious in rabies-infected rodents. In 1972, a study on rabid squirrels showed that half of the infected animals that died of rabies showed no clinical signs [29,30].

Two cases of rabies in domestic rabbits (*Oryctolagus cuniculus*) in Maryland in 1999 are worthy of note here. In both of these cases, rabbits were sent home with their owners after examination and the owners were instructed to hand- or force-feed the rabbits, which later died and were found to be rabid. Clinical signs of illness in these rabbits on examination included weakness in forelimbs, palpable subcutaneous crepitus, slight intermittent head tremors, ear infection, nasal discharge, and anorexia. On readmission, one rabbit exhibited heavy wheezing, inability to stand, head tilt, and bilateral conjunctivitis. The disease course culminated in a recumbent and nonresponsive state. The case history of this rabbit included an attack by a raccoon in a rabies-endemic area, resulting in a wound to the ear and the rabbit being covered in saliva [31]. It is critical that rabies be considered in the differential diagnosis of any rabbit coming into contact with raccoons, especially those rabbits displaying neurologic signs. Furthermore, discharging an animal that has been exposed to potentially rabid wildlife should be avoided, as should recommending owners to force-feed these animals, bringing them into closer contact to a potentially rabid pet.

Despite natural infection of rabbits being rare, it is imperative to remember that rabbits are used for rabies diagnostic testing and were used for creation of the first rabies vaccine by Louis Pasteur in the 1880s. Rabbits are highly susceptible to rabies virus infection, have incubation periods between 2 and 3 weeks after intracerebral inoculation, and usually develop paralytic rabies. Experimentally infected rabbits display anorexia, fever, restlessness, weight loss, and such neurologic signs as teeth grinding, head tremors, poor coordination of the hind limbs, and ascending paralysis. The affected rabbit usually dies within 3 to 4 days [31]. Veterinarians should advise patients that no rabies vaccine is available for rabbits; thus, prevention is essential. Rabbits should be kept indoors or kept in elevated hutches without exposed wire mesh floors, and rabbits should be supervised at all times when exercising outdoors [31].

LABORATORY DIAGNOSIS FOR ANIMAL RABIES

Clinical signs are good indications for rabies in small animals. Rapid and accurate laboratory diagnosis for animal rabies is important for confirmation, however. In addition, many animals may not show typical signs of rabies. Usually, rabid or suspected rabid wild animals are road kill or otherwise deceased when brought into diagnostic laboratories.

Laboratory diagnosis is important because it provides not only data for epidemiologic investigation of animal rabies but guidance for initiation of PEP in affected people [32].

Direct Florescent Antibody Assay

The most frequently used method for rabies diagnosis in the laboratory is the direct fluorescent antibody assay (dFA) [33–35]. Usually, brain smears or brain imprints from rabid or suspected rabid animals are reacted with fluorescein isothiocyanate (FITC)–conjugated anti-rabies N antibodies [33,36]. When observed under a fluorescent microscope, the green-fluorescent foci show the rabies virus antigen (Fig. 3A). The dFA is rapid, economic, and sensitive for laboratory diagnosis of animal rabies. Rabies antigens can be detected by the specific antibody; however, they should be differentiated from the nonspecific background.

Direct Rapid Immunohistochemistry Test

Recently, the Centers for Disease Control and Prevention (CDC) developed the direct rapid immunohistochemistry test (dRIT) [37], which is similar to the dFA. Brain smears or imprints on glass slides are fixed with 10% buffered formalin [37]. According to standard immunohistochemical staining, the virus antigen can be detected by anti-rabies N monoclonal antibody and examined under a light microscope. The sensitivity and specificity of the dRIT are equivalent to those of the dFA [37].

Virus Isolation

Mouse inoculation is a World Health Organization (WHO)–recommended method to confirm the findings of the dFA when the result is negative

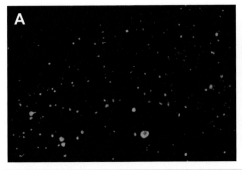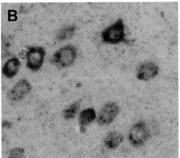

Fig. 3. Detection of rabies virus antigens by dFA (A) and immunohistochemistry (B). (A) Virus foci show positive stains with green-fluorescent color. (*From* Centers for Disease Control and Prevention. Rabies diagnosis. Available at: http://www.cdc.gov/rabies/diagnosis.html. Accessed September 20, 2007.) (B) The paraffin-embedded slide was stained by anti-rabies virus nucleoprotein monoclonal antibody 802–2. Rabies antigens in the cytoplasm and inclusions are shown in brown (using diaminobenzidine as the substance), and the cell nuclei are shown in blue.

[38,39]. Usually, brain suspension or spinal fluid from rabid or suspected rabid animals is intracerebrally inoculated into mouse brain. Two mice are sacrificed every 2 days after infection until day 20, and brain smears are subjected to the dFA. The 50% mouse intracerebral lethal dose ($MICLD_{50}$) can be calculated [40]. Virus isolation can also be performed in cell culture, usually on neuroblastoma cells [41]. Using this method, the 50% tissue culture infective dose ($TCID_{50}$) can be calculated [40]. Cell culture inoculation is as sensitive as the mouse inoculation test [42], and it requires less time to obtain results.

Reverse Transcriptase Polymerase Chain Reaction

Reverse transcriptase polymerase chain reaction (RT-PCR) is a newly developed method for rabies diagnosis [33,43]. RT-PCR is useful when the sample size is small, such as when collecting saliva and spinal fluid. Viral RNA is amplified by RT-PCR with primers usually designed from the N gene, the most conserved gene in rabies virus. RT-PCR for rabies diagnosis is as rapid as the dFA and is as sensitive as the mouse inoculation test [44]. RT-PCR is also widely used in epidemiologic investigation and outbreak studies. When combined with sequencing, this method can also be used to differentiate rabies virus variants from multiple species of animals [17,43,45,46]. Viral variants can also be differentiated with different monoclonal antibodies in an indirect fluorescent antibody assay [17,47].

Histopathology and Immunohistochemistry

Rabies diagnosis in small animals can also be performed on brain tissues by histopathologic examination and immunohistochemistry [48]. Histopathologic examination may show lymphocytic inflammation, perivascular cuffing, gliosis, and neurodegeneration [49]. Inflammation is diffuse in neuraxis. The parenchymal glial response is at first microglial but later mixed with astrocytes.

Neuron degeneration is often not severe [50]. The severity of inflammation may vary between animal species. Sometimes, a spongiform encephalopathy with vacuolation in the gray matter can be observed [51]. Negri bodies, which are ovoid eosinophilic intracytoplasmic inclusions [52,53], are a hallmark for rabies diagnosis. Yet, Negri bodies are not found in all rabies cases [49].

In fixed-brain tissue, immunohistochemistry can be used to confirm the diagnosis (Fig. 3B).

By using the rabies-specific antibody and avidin-biotin colorimetric detection system, the virus can be detected. Antigen-positive neurons can be found in the brain and spinal cord.

Detection of Rabies Virus–Specific Antibodies

Detection of specific antibodies can be used as diagnostic tools for rabies. There are many methods that have been developed to detect rabies-specific antibodies. The RFFIT is the method used most often to detect virus-neutralizing antibodies [33,54]. ELISA has also been used to detect virus-specific antibodies when the ELISA plate is coated with rabies virus antigens [55,56]. Because antibodies take several days to develop, this method is rarely used in diagnosis of animal rabies. Rather, detection of virus-specific antibodies is often used in vaccination studies.

Rabies Control in Domestic Small Animals

Rabies control in small animals is by routine immunization with inactivated rabies virus vaccines, which have been approved for dogs, cats, and ferrets. First vaccination is performed at 3 months of age and is followed by a booster 1 year later. Subsequent immunization is performed annually or triennially depending on the type of vaccines used [57]. Recently, a recombinant canarypox vaccine has been licensed for cats with a similar immunization schedule [58]. Currently, it is required by law that dogs and cats be vaccinated against rabies.

SUMMARY

Rabies in small animals has been dramatically reduced in the United States since the introduction of rabies vaccination of domestic animals in the 1940s. As a consequence, the number of human rabies cases has declined to only a couple per year. During the past several years, the dog rabies variant has almost disappeared completely. Rabies in wildlife has skyrocketed, however. At the present, there are many concurrent rabies epizootics in wildlife in the United States: raccoon rabies along the eastern seaboard, skunk rabies in the central states and California, Arctic fox rabies in Alaska, and red and gray fox rabies in the southwestern states. In addition, bat rabies is endemic in the 48 contiguous states. Each wildlife species carries its own rabies variant(s). These wildlife epizootics present a constant public health threat in addition to the danger of reintroducing rabies to domestic animals. Vaccination is the key to prevent rabies in small animals and rabies transmission to human beings.

References

[1] Fu ZF. Rabies and rabies research: past, present and future. Vaccine 1997;(Suppl 15): S20–4.

[2] Meslin FX. [Current situation on human rabies control and anti-rabies vaccination]. Sante 1994;4:203–4 [in French].

[3] Meslin FX, Fishbein DB, Matter HC. Rationale and prospects for rabies elimination in developing countries. Curr Top Microbiol Immunol 1994;187:1–26.

[4] Noah DL, Drenzek CL, Smith JS, et al. Epidemiology of human rabies in the United States, 1980 to 1996. Ann Intern Med 1998;128:922–30.

[5] Blanton JD, Hanlon CA, Rupprecht CE. Rabies surveillance in the United States during 2006. J Am Vet Med Assoc 2007;231:540–56.

[6] Blanton JD, Krebs JW, Hanlon CA, et al. Rabies surveillance in the United States during 2005. J Am Vet Med Assoc 2006;229:1897–911.

[7] Real LA, Russell C, Waller L, et al. Spatial dynamics and molecular ecology of North American rabies. J Hered 2005;96:253–60.

[8] Childs JE, Curns AT, Dey ME, et al. Predicting the local dynamics of epizootic rabies among raccoons in the United States. Proc Natl Acad Sci U S A 2000;97:13666–71.

[9] Biek R, Henderson JC, Waller LA, et al. A high-resolution genetic signature of demographic and spatial expansion in epizootic rabies virus. Proc Natl Acad Sci U S A 2007;104:7993–8.

[10] Charlton KM, Webster WA, Casey GA, et al. Skunk rabies. Rev Infect Dis 1988;(10 Suppl 4):S626–8.

[11] Guerra MA, Curns AT, Rupprecht CE, et al. Skunk and raccoon rabies in the eastern United States: temporal and spatial analysis. Emerg Infect Dis 2003;9:1143–50.

[12] Leslie MJ, Messenger S, Rohde RE, et al. Bat-associated rabies virus in skunks. Emerg Infect Dis 2006;12:1274–7.

[13] Ballard WB, Follmann EH, Ritter DG, et al. Rabies and canine distemper in an Arctic fox population in Alaska. J Wildl Dis 2001;37:133–7.

[14] Carey AB. The ecology of red foxes, gray foxes, and rabies in the Eastern United States. Wildlife Society Bulletin 1982;10:18–26.

[15] Clark KA, Neill SU, Smith JS, et al. Epizootic canine rabies transmitted by coyotes in south Texas. J Am Vet Med Assoc 1994;204:536–40.

[16] Gordon ER, Curns AT, Krebs JW, et al. Temporal dynamics of rabies in a wildlife host and the risk of cross-species transmission. Epidemiol Infect 2004;132:515–24.

[17] McQuiston JH, Yager PA, Smith JS, et al. Epidemiologic characteristics of rabies virus variants in dogs and cats in the United States, 1999. J Am Vet Med Assoc 2001;218: 1939–42.

[18] Rabies. In: What every dog owner should know about rabies. Available at: http://www.canismajor.com/dog/rabies.html. Accessed February 2, 2008

[19] Barlough JE, Scott FW, Richards JR. Max's house rabies. Available at: http://maxshouse.com/rabies.htm. Accessed February 2, 2008

[20] Barnes HL, Chrisman CL, Farina L, et al. Clinical evaluation of rabies virus meningoencephalomyelitis in a dog. J Am Anim Hosp Assoc 2003;39:547–50.

[21] Suja MS, Mahadevan A, Madhusudana SN, et al. Cerebral cysticercosis mimicking rabies in a dog. Vet Rec 2003;153:304–5.

[22] Nichols PR, Morris DO, Beale KM. A retrospective study of canine and feline cutaneous vasculitis. Vet Dermatol 2001;12:255–64.

[23] Krebs JW, Rupprecht CE, Childs JE. Rabies surveillance in the United States during 1999. J Am Vet Med Assoc 2000;217:1799–811.

[24] Jackson AC, Wunner WH, editors. Rabies. 2nd edition. London (UK): Academic Press; 2007. p. 221–2.

[25] Tepsumethanon V, Lumlertdacha B, Mitmoonpitak C, et al. Survival of naturally infected rabid dogs and cats. Clin Infect Dis 2004;39:278–80.

[26] Ryland LM, Bernard SL, Gorham JR, et al, editors. A clinical guide to the pet ferret. In: Practical exotic animal medicine. Trenton (NJ): Veterinary learning systems; 1997. p. 122–9,155.

[27] Niezgoda M, Briggs DJ, Shaddock J, et al. Pathogenesis of experimentally induced rabies in domestic ferrets. Am J Vet Res 1997;58:1327–31.

[28] Niezgoda M, Briggs DJ, Shaddock J, et al. Viral excretion in domestic ferrets (Mustela putorius furo) inoculated with a raccoon rabies isolate. Am J Vet Res 1998;59:1629–32.

[29] Eidson M, Matthews SD, Willsey AL, et al. Rabies virus infection in a pet guinea pig and seven pet rabbits. J Am Vet Med Assoc 2005;227:932–5.

[30] Winkler WG. Rodent rabies. In: Baer GM, editor. The natural history of rabies. 2nd edition. Boca Raton (FL): CRC Press, INC; 1991. p. 405–10.

[31] Karp BE, Ball NE, Scott CR, et al. Rabies in two privately owned domestic rabbits. J Am Vet Med Assoc 1999;215:1824–7,1806.

[32] CDC. First human death associated with raccoon rabies—Virginia, 2003. MMWR Morb Mortal Wkly Rep 2003;52:1102–3.

[33] Rabies—bulletin—Europe. In: Rabies information system of the WHO Collaboration Centre for Rabies Surveillance and Research. Available at: http://www.who-rabies-bulletin.org/About_Rabies/Diagnosis.aspx. Accessed September 20, 2007.

[34] Dean DJ, Ableseth MK. Laboratory techniques in rabies: the fluorescent antibody test. Monograph Series. World Health Organization 1973;23:73–84.

[35] Dean DJ, Ableseth MK, Atanasiu P. Laboratory techniques in rabies. 4th edition. Geneva (IL): World Health Organization; 1966.

[36] Trimarchi CV, Debbie JG. Standardization and quantitation of immunofluorescence in the rabies fluorescent-antibody test. Appl Microbiol 1972;24:609–12.

[37] Lembo T, Niezgoda M, Velasco-Villa A, et al. Evaluation of a direct, rapid immunohistochemical test for rabies diagnosis. Emerg Infect Dis 2006;12:310–3.

[38] Koprowski H. Laboratory techniques in rabies: the mouse inoculation test. Monogr Ser World Health Organ 1973;23:85–9.

[39] Webster WA, Casey GA, Charlton KM. The mouse inoculation test in rabies diagnosis: early diagnosis in mice during the incubation period. Can J Comp Med 1976;40:322–5.

[40] Reed L, Muench H. A simple method of estimating fifty percent endpoints. Am J Hyg 1938;27:493–7.

[41] Zanoni R, Hornlimann B, Wandeler AI, et al. Rabies tissue culture infection test as an alternative for the mouse inoculation test. ALTEX 1990;7:15–23.

[42] Rudd RJ, Trimarchi CV. Development and evaluation of an in vitro virus isolation procedure as a replacement for the mouse inoculation test in rabies diagnosis. J Clin Microbiol 1989;27:2522–8.

[43] Sacramento D, Bourhy H, Tordo N. PCR technique as an alternative method for diagnosis and molecular epidemiology of rabies virus. Mol Cell Probes 1991;5:229–40.

[44] Macedo CI, Carnieli P Jr, Brandao PE, et al. Diagnosis of human rabies cases by polymerase chain reaction of neck-skin samples. Braz J Infect Dis 2006;10:341–5.

[45] Crepin P, Audry L, Rotivel Y, et al. Intravitam diagnosis of human rabies by PCR using saliva and cerebrospinal fluid. J Clin Microbiol 1998;36:1117–21.

[46] Tordo N, Sacramento D, Bourhy H. Laboratory techniques in rabies. 4th edition. Geneva (IL): World Health Organization; 1996.

[47] Dean DJ, Ableseth MK, Atanasiu P. Laboratory techniques in rabies. 4th edition. Geneva (IL): World Health Organization; 1996.

[48] Palmer DG, Ossent P, Suter MM, et al. Demonstration of rabies viral antigen in paraffin tissue sections: comparison of the immunofluorescence technique with the unlabeled antibody enzyme method. Am J Vet Res 1985;46:283–6.

[49] Summers BA, Cummings JF, deLahunta A. Veterinary neuropathology. St. Louis (MO): Mosby; 1994. p. 95–9.

[50] Rupprecht CE, Dietzschold B. Perspectives on rabies virus pathogenesis. Lab Invest 1987;57:603–6.

[51] Charlton KM, Casey GA, Webster WA, et al. Experimental rabies in skunks and foxes. Pathogenesis of the spongiform lesions. Lab Invest 1987;57:634–45.

[52] Butts JD, Bouldin TW, Walker DH. Morphological characteristics of a unique intracytoplasmic neuronal inclusion body. Acta Neuropathol (Berl) 1984;62:345–7.

[53] Yang LM, Zhao LZ, Hu RL, et al. A novel double-antigen sandwich enzyme-linked immunosorbent assay for measurement of antibodies against rabies virus. Clin Vaccine Immunol 2006;13:966–8.

[54] Budzko DB, Charamella LJ, Jelinek D, et al. Rapid test for detection of rabies antibodies in human serum. J Clin Microbiol 1983;17:481–4.

[55] Mebatsion T, Frost JW, Krauss H. Enzyme-linked immunosorbent assay (ELISA) using staphylococcal protein A for the measurement of rabies antibody in various species. Zentralbl Veterinarmed B 1989;36:532–6.

[56] Mebatsion T, Sillero-Zubiri C, Gottelli D, et al. Detection of rabies antibody by ELISA and RFFIT in unvaccinated dogs and in the endangered Simien jackal (Canis simensis) of Ethiopia. Zentralbl Veterinarmed B 1992;39:233–5.

[57] Compendium of animal rabies prevention and control, 2000. The National Association of State Public Health Veterinarians. J Am Vet Med Assoc 2000;216:338–43.

[58] Compendium of animal rabies prevention and control, 2006. J Am Vet Med Assoc 2006;228:858–64.

Vet Clin Small Anim 38 (2008) 863–878

VETERINARY CLINICS
SMALL ANIMAL PRACTICE

Emerging Viral Encephalitides in Dogs and Cats

Bradley L. Njaa, DVM, MVSc

Department of Veterinary Pathobiology, Center for Veterinary Health Sciences, Oklahoma State University, 226 McElroy Hall, Stillwater, OK 74078, USA

Viral encephalitides in dogs and cats have a long history. Rabies, denoted for many centuries as primarily a canine disease, is the first zoonotic disease studied, and investigations of this virus ultimately led to the discovery of protective vaccination and postexposure prophylaxis. Long before the germ theory came into being, there were numerous documented accounts of dogs described as being "mad," "vicious," or full of "rage" that terrorized regions of Europe and France causing fatal "hydrophobia" in bitten human beings [1]. Over the many centuries that followed, canids were tagged with the distinction of spreading this scourge among other canids in addition to human beings. By the early 1820s, rabies would be the first zoonotic disease to become the focus of intense comparative medicine research [1]. Thankfully, it became a prototype disease studied by Louis Pasteur and others in the late nineteenth century and early twentieth century that led to the development of crude but effective vaccines that would eventually protect people and animals from this disease [1].

The second most common cause of encephalitis in dogs is canine distemper virus (CDV). Fortunately for human beings, this is not a zoonotic pathogen, but CDV devastated the canine population in the mid-1900s. Relief from CDV came with the development of effective vaccines. Separate articles within this issue are dedicated to canine distemper virus and rabies virus.

In these two encephalitic viruses, there is variable morbidity, with mortality rates reaching 100% with rabies virus. Recently, there has been a return to the zoonotic intersection of viral pathogens affecting dogs, cats, and people. In contrast to rabies virus and CDV, the viral pathogens described in this article are emerging pathogens. Infections in dogs and cats by these emerging viruses are associated with low morbidity and low mortality. Dogs and cats are believed to be dead-end hosts for the pathogens discussed in this article. In some cases, however, dogs or cats may represent sentinel species for possible transmission to human beings.

E-mail address: brad.njaa@okstate.edu

0195-5616/08/$ – see front matter
doi:10.1016/j.cvsm.2008.03.006

WEST NILE VIRUS

First isolated from a human being with febrile disease in the late 1930s in the West Nile District of Uganda in Africa, West Nile Virus (WNV) was known to cause sporadic disease outbreaks in various parts of Africa, Europe, Asia, and Australia [2,3]. In the late summer and autumn of 1999, WNV emerged in North America for the first time, causing deaths in birds, horses, and people in New York City and several surrounding states [4]. Based on phylogenetic analysis, one or more of the viruses isolated and sequenced from the epicenter were most closely related to a sequenced virus that had been isolated from an outbreak of initially unexplained deaths in geese in Israel in 1997 and 1998 [4–7]. The transmission of the Israel strain to the United States remains a mystery. Possible theories include accidental importation of mosquitoes from endemic regions of the Middle East and illegal importation of geese from the outbreak region [5].

Initial reports of WNV outbreaks were primarily nonfatal febrile illnesses in people and birds until the early to mid-1960s, when encephalitic disease was reported in people and horses infected with WNV in Egypt and France [8]. In the 1990s, there were increased reports of human disease implicating WNV. These reports were often accompanied by fatal illness in horse and bird populations [8]. With the exception of one early report of encephalitic disease in a dog from Botswana in 1977, reports of natural infection with WNV in dogs or cats did not appear in the literature until 1999 and later [9–15].

WNV is an arbovirus in the family Flaviviridae, genus *Flavivirus*, and antigenic complex Japanese encephalitis virus (JEV) group [3]. It is maintained in a geographic location by cycling between ornithophilic mosquitoes, primarily of the genus *Culex*, and wild birds in the region. Human beings, horses, and other vertebrates, such as dogs and cats, are incidental hosts. WNV is further classified into phylogenetically distinct lineages that are essentially geographic segregations and are based on signature amino acid variations in envelope proteins [3,8]. Lineage 1 viruses are found in North Africa, Europe, Asia, the Americas, and Australia, whereas lineage 2 viruses are found exclusively in southern Africa and Madagascar [16]. All the North American WNV isolates are lineage 1 viruses. As a group, lineage 1 viruses are more neuroinvasive and have a greater tendency to cause more severe encephalitic disease than lineage 2 viruses. Neuroinvasive lineage 2 viruses have been identified, however [8,16]. The genetic determinants for virulence and neuroinvasiveness have yet to be definitively identified. All the canine and feline cases of natural disease leading to encephalitis have been attributable to lineage 1 viral infections, with the exception of a single case in a dog in South Africa that was initially reported as Wesselsbron disease but later confirmed as WNV [9–15].

Although initially identified in North America in northeastern states (New York, Connecticut, New Jersey, and Maryland) in 1999, WNV has subsequently spread through North America and has become endemic [17,18]. Based on surveillance data published on-line by the US and Canadian governments, WNV activity has been documented in humans or animals and mosquitoes in all the lower 48 states and in 7 Canadian provinces. As of the end of 2007, the provinces and states with the highest per capita incidence of WNV activity are as follows: Saskatchewan, Manitoba, and Alberta in Canada and South Dakota, North Dakota, Wyoming, New Mexico, Mississippi, Nebraska, Louisiana, and Colorado in the United States [19,20].

Surveillance Data for Dogs and Cats

Limited studies have documented the seroprevalence of neutralizing antibodies to WNV in dogs and cats. There are primarily five published studies addressing the percentage of surveyed dogs in a given region that have serum neutralizing antibodies to WNV [4,11,21–23]. The regions assessed include two areas in South Africa, portions of New York City during the initial introduction of WNV to North America, two regions in Louisiana a few years after its introduction to North America, and Turkey. The range of seropositivity in North American dogs varies from a low of 3% (5 of 169) of dogs in Missouri in 2002 to 5.3% (10 of 189) of dogs in New York City at the time of introduction to 26% (116 of 442) of dogs in Louisiana during the summer and fall of 2002. Not surprisingly, in Kile and colleagues' study [22], outdoor dogs had 19 times greater odds of being seropositive than indoor dogs and stray dogs had nearly twice greater odds of being seropositive than family-owned dogs. Dogs from the South African study and the later Turkey study had higher seroprevalence: 37% (138 of 377 dogs) and 37.7% (43 of 114 dogs), respectively.

Seroconversion in cats has also been studied, but the results are much different. In two of the three surveys, none of the cats in Turkey or the New York City area had serum neutralizing antibodies to WNV [4,23]. In the third study in Louisiana, only 9% (13 of 138) of cats had serum neutralizing antibodies to WNV [22].

Natural Disease

There are few reported cases of disease attributable to WNV infections in dogs. Included in this group are 5 dogs and a wolf puppy [9–13]. Additionally, there was an immunohistochemical (IHC) study that evaluated encephalitic brain tissue from dogs and cats of unknown cause using antibodies specific for numerous neuroinvasive pathogens and found WNV antigen staining in 5 of 53 dogs examined [14]. In the latter study, clinical data are general to the population and limited to what was provided at the time of necropsy.

The most frequently reported clinical findings are fever, ataxia, and depression. Temperatures ranged from 40.3° to 42.2°C. Other common findings included anorexia, weakness, diarrhea of variable severity, conscious proprioceptive deficits, and altered mentation. Ocular discharge has been rarely reported. Animals became profoundly weak and unable to rise. Rarely, episodic and uncontrolled rolling progressed to whole-body tremors that were unresponsive to oral phenobarbital therapy [12]. Most of the dogs infected with WNV are humanely euthanatized because of the poor prognosis given.

Reports in cats are more scant. Early publications of WNV affecting cats were initially presented on Web sites that have not been maintained. A New

York City Web site created during the initial WNV outbreak documented three cases in cats whereby WNV was isolated as referenced by Karaca and colleagues [24]. Only one of those cases is documented elsewhere by Komar [15] as a cat from New Jersey that was euthanatized for seizures. Although the virus was isolated from the brain, details of histologic examination were not reported. The only other reference to natural disease in cats is the IHC report by Schwab and colleagues [14] in which 12% (4 of 33) of cats with non-suppurative meningoencephalitis stained positively for WNV antigen. Clinical signs reported were vague, however.

Experimental Disease

Dogs can be infected with WNV by subcutaneous, intravenous, intracerebral, intranasal, or intracardiac inoculation [21,24]. Natural infection is presumed to be inoculation by infected mosquitoes, however. Most recent publications have provided convincing evidence that dogs can be infected by allowing infected mosquitoes to feed on susceptible dogs [24–26]. In every instance, none of the infected dogs developed clinical signs of disease. Yet, nearly all the dogs developed viremia and detectable neutralizing antibodies to WNV for a variable amount of time after inoculation.

Two studies looked at experimental infections in cats. In both studies, cats were inoculated with WNV by infected mosquitoes [24,25]. In addition, Austgen and colleagues [25] included a group of cats that were infected by ingesting mice that had been infected with WNV. Only 2 cats out of an aggregate of 41 cats developed a period of cyclical pyrexia, and a total of 3 cats were initially lethargic after challenge. No cat in any of the experiments developed neurologic signs, however. As was observed in the dogs, most of the naive cats developed neutralizing antibodies to WNV and developed a short-lived but measurable viremia.

Gross and Histologic Pathology Findings

Of all the animals studied, only one dog had gross evidence of disease related to WNV infection, namely, fibrinous epicarditis [10]. This is thought to be related to myocarditis, which often accompanies WNV infections in various species, including dogs.

Histologic lesions associated with WNV infections are localized to the brain and heart. Within the brain of affected animals is a mild to moderate, primarily lymphocytic to lymphohistiocytic (nonsuppurative) perivascular infiltrate with lymphocytic, histiocytic, and, occasionally, neutrophilic encephalitis, which primarily affects the gray matter. Neuronal necrosis, glial nodule formation in the neuropil, and variable degrees of meningitis can also be seen [10–14]. Most of these cases are described as predominantly gray matter disease with variable involvement of the white matter. In one wolf and one dog, a focal area of malacia was reported in each. In the wolf brain, there was an area of malacia associated with foamy macrophage infiltration within the basal nuclei [10], whereas in the dog, a medullary lesion at the level of the olivary nucleus contained an area of malacia and necrosis with fibrinous effusion, hemorrhages, clusters of infiltrating foamy macrophages, and many swollen axons [12]. One dog had an area of severe hippocampal malacia suggestive of antemortem seizure activity [14].

Myocardial lesions in affected animals comprise variable numbers of degenerate to necrotic hypereosinophilic myocytes with loss of striation and loss of nuclear detail. Variable numbers of predominantly lymphocytes and histiocytes with fewer neutrophils infiltrate the surrounding interstitium [10,11,13]. Occasionally, there were hemorrhages and vasculitis in the areas of most severe inflammation and necrosis [13].

In the rare cases described in cats, gross lesions have not been reported and histologic changes were restricted to the brain [14]. Of the four cats described, two had moderate to severe meningoencephalitis involving the gray and white matter, one had mild lymphocytic polioencephalitis and moderate lymphohistiocytic meningitis with severe vacuolization of the cerebral white matter, and a fourth had severe focal fibrinopurulent meningitis. This last cat described also had severe acute neuronal necrosis of the hippocampus, suggestive of antemortem seizure activity.

Diagnosis
Because the fatality rate of reported cases in dogs and cats is so high, confirmation of a diagnosis of WNV infection can make use of multiple modalities. Clinical signs in concert with histologic lesions involving the gray and white matter and myocardial necrosis and inflammation are highly suggestive of WNV infection. Definitive confirmation uses molecular diagnostic techniques, such as IHC and reverse transcriptase polymerase chain reaction (RT-PCR). Isolation of virus using vero cells is the most commonly reported method of isolating WNV.

Prevention and Control
As was determined by a seroprevalence study, minimizing exposure of dogs and cats to infected mosquitoes resulted in a 19 times odds reduction of becoming infected [22]. Thus, insect repellants are likely to have some positive effect in minimizing exposure. In addition, there is a recent publication validating the efficacy and safety of a canarypox-vectored WNV vaccine for the protection of dogs and cats against mosquited WNV challenge [24]. In light of the relatively low seroprevalence in dogs and extremely low presence of antibodies in cats, in addition to the relative paucity of reported cases of fatal encephalitic WNV infections in dogs and cats, however, it is unlikely that routine vaccination is warranted.

HENIPAVIRUSES
Henipaviruses are a recently described genus of the family Paramyxoviridae in the subfamily Paramyxoviridae that have recently emerged as a cause for zoonotic disease spilling over from flying foxes [27]. Originally, an equine Morbillivirus (now referred to as Hendra virus after the original location where it first appeared) was the cause of a severe respiratory disease outbreak in horses in

Brisbane, Queensland in the late fall of 1994 [28–30]. More than 60% of affected horses died, and 1 human being died. Nipah virus was first described in Malaysia in late autumn of 1998 as a cause of febrile and respiratory disease in weaner and growing pigs and an often fatal encephalitic disease in exposed pig farm workers and abattoir workers [31]. Initially, little was known about these viruses, and pathogenesis studies were undertaken to determine which species were susceptible. Early in these studies, it was determined that cats were highly susceptible, whereas dogs were highly resistant to henipaviruses [32]. Virus was isolated from the brain from one of the two cats experimentally inoculated subcutaneously with Hendra virus. Although there are no reports of natural infection by these viruses causing encephalitic disease, there is ample experimental evidence that only the Nipah virus is capable of causing severe encephalitic and meningeal disease in cats.

Surveillance Data of Dogs and Cats
After the discovery that cats were highly susceptible to Hendra virus, an extensive serologic survey was performed and none of the sera from 500 cats in metropolitan Brisbane had detectable antibodies to the virus [32]. The initial publication describing the first outbreak of Nipah virus in Malaysia briefly alludes to the fact that serologic studies confirmed that the virus was circulating among dogs and cats in the outbreak area [31]. A single cat and dog are documented in the report as having been infected with isolates that were genetically identical to original Nipah virus isolates obtained from the original outbreak. No other information is provided about these cases, however. In another study, sick or dying dogs were included as a possible risk factor in a case-control study, but there are no data reported that confirm the vague signs of unsteady gait, loss of appetite, and frothing at the mouth in these dogs were attributable to Nipah virus infection [33]. Finally, testing the theory that cats may come into direct contact with the reservoir host, fruit bats of the genus *Pteropus*, 32 feral cats were captured within a 200-m radius of a known bat colony in Air Batang and all were negative for neutralizing antibodies to Nipah virus [34]. The investigators' proposed explanation for these findings includes rare exposure to Nipah virus in nature, case fatality rate so high that most cats die rather than develop immunity, or too small a sample size.

Clinical Disease
Natural infections in dogs and cats are poorly documented. Hooper and colleagues [35] describe rare instances of naturally occurring *Henipavirus* infections in cats and dogs. Natural Hendra virus infections in cats were not reported, but experimental infections resulted in severe pulmonary disease necessitating humane euthanasia early in the course of clinical disease [36]. In the original subcutaneous inoculation study, infected cats became inappetent with increased respiratory rates by 5 to 6 days and died 1 day later [32]. Only one natural case of Nipah virus infection in a cat exists to date that was confirmed by necropsy [35]. The reported clinical sign was severe dyspnea. In experimental cases of Nipah virus, clinical signs were also attributed to severe pulmonary

edema and hydrothorax. Signs attributable to neurologic disease have not been reported, however.

Natural infections in dogs are reported only with Nipah virus infections. Two dogs with active disease were reported [35,37]. One dog was reportedly febrile with signs of respiratory distress, conjunctivitis, and mucopurulent ocular and nasal discharge. This animal eventually became moribund. A second dog was found dead. Both dogs were from a village in which active Nipah viral infections had occurred in regional pig farms.

Gross and Histologic Pathology Findings

No cats thus far that have been naturally or experimentally infected with Hendra virus have developed signs of or histologic evidence of encephalitis [38]. Cats infected with Nipah virus have developed lesions in the central nervous system (CNS), however [35,39]. Documented lesions included nonsuppurative meningitis with rare infiltrating neutrophils, meningeal vasculitis with endothelial cell syncytial formation, and extension of the inflammation into the adjacent neural parenchyma at optic tracts in one cat.

During the outbreaks of Nipah virus infections in Malaysia in 1998, sick and dying dogs were considered a possible risk factor for the development of encephalitic disease in people, but the disease and pathogen in dogs are poorly documented [33]. One dog was reportedly showing signs resembling infection with CDV [35]. Histologic examination revealed nonsuppurative meningitis with ischemic rarefaction in the brain and cerebral vascular degeneration.

Diagnosis

These viruses can be grown by a wide range of cell culture systems, including cells derived from mammalian species and birds, reptiles, amphibians, and fish [32]. Cell culture monolayers develop characteristic syncytial cell formation and cytopathogenic effect (CPE). Early in the outbreaks, PCR primers were generated from consensus *Paramyxoviridae* matrix proteins [28]. There are immunohistochemical stains available for identification of virus in formalin-fixed tissue samples.

Prevention and Control

CNS disease in cats and dogs infected with henipaviruses is an exceedingly rare event. Thus, it is highly unlikely that vaccines are going to be developed to protect naive cats and dogs. Minimizing exposure to the urine and body fluids of flying foxes, especially when they are pregnant, likely minimizes the chances of developing neutralizing antibodies or disease.

HIGHLY PATHOGENIC H5N1 AVIAN INFLUENZA VIRUS

Highly pathogenic avian influenza (HPAI) virus was thought to be a pathogen that could devastate affected countries because of trade restrictions and lost income associated with dead poultry. In 1997, however, Asia would become the epicenter for an outbreak of HPAI H5N1 virus in poultry that crossed presumed species barriers, causing disease and death in human beings and possibly other mammals [40]. The zoonotic potential of HPAI then became a major concern. A second Asian outbreak of HPAI H5N1 virus infection in poultry occurred in late 2003 and early 2004 in which mortality rates were extremely high. Case fatality rates approached 50% in human cases [41]. During this same outbreak, it became apparent that other mammals were susceptible, namely, cats, and that they may serve as a source of virus for human beings.

Avian influenza virus is in the genus influenza type A virus in the family Orthomyxoviridae. Influenza type A viruses are further subtyped based on the antigenic variation of two surface glycoproteins; hemagglutinin (H) and neuraminidase (N) [42]. There are currently 15 different H and 9 different N subtypes, and combinations of all circulate in avian species. Originally called "fowl plague," HPAI viruses are designated as highly virulent based on the type and sequence of amino acids and the type of carbohydrate found in the cleavage site of H glycoproteins, thereby determining the relative ease of cleavability by proteases at this cleavage site. Currently, virulent strains of influenza type A are confined to H5 and H7 subtypes.

During the second HPAI H5N1 virus outbreak in Southeast Asia, suspicious deaths occurred in zoo cats in late 2003 and in a domestic cat in early 2004 [43,44]. What was unusual about these deaths is that although the illness began as a febrile and respiratory process, it quickly progressed to a systemic disease with evidence of encephalitis. Thus, not only did HPAI H5N1 virus cross the species barrier from avian to feline species, but it raised the alarm that H5N1 virus could possibly be transmitted from infected cats to unsuspecting owners or zookeepers.

Serologic Evidence of Disease in Dogs and Cats

After the second Asian outbreak of HPAI H5N1 virus in 2005, a virologist at the National Institute of Animal Health in Bangkok undertook a serologic survey of dogs and cats in the area [45]. A total of 626 village dogs and 111 cats were tested for the presence of antibodies to H5N1 in the Suphan Buri district of central Thailand. Just more than 25% (160 of 626) of dogs and 7% (8 of 111) of cats were positive for antibodies to H5N1. An Austrian study analyzed blood samples from a group of cats that had been exposed to infected birds at the same shelter, and over the course of 50 days after exposure, only 2 cats tested positive for antibodies to H5N1. A definite denominator is not clear, because quarantined cats that repeatedly tested negative were adopted from the shelter [46]. More recently, researchers in Milan, Italy tested 196 cats, and all were negative for antibodies to H5N1 [47].

Natural Disease

There are a small number of reports of natural infections causing disease in wild and domestic cats, [43,44,46,48,49] and one documenting natural infection in a dog [50]. To date, lesions of encephalitic disease have only been documented in cats and do not occur in infected dogs.

Affected cats initially had high fevers, recorded as high as 41°C in a domestic cat, and experienced respiratory distress [44]. The disease course progressed to depression, convulsions, and ataxia by 2 days after the onset of disease in the domestic cat. In the four large cats, death was "unexpected" in the zoo in Suphanburi, Thailand [43,44]. In an outbreak that occurred 10 months later in a zoo in Sriracha, Chonburi, Thailand, 16 tigers, ranging in age from 6 to 24 months, initially developed high fevers and had respiratory distress [48]. Three days after first observed clinical signs, the sick tigers were dead, having developed neurologic signs and all expressing a serosanguineous nasal discharge. Laboratory findings in this latter group included severe leukopenia and thrombocytopenia and elevations in alanine aminotransferase (ALT) and aspartate aminotransferase (AST).

In all these cases, there had been exposure to avian species before the outbreak. Fresh poultry from a local abattoir fed to the four zoo cats was presumed to be the source of H5N1 [43]. The one domestic cat that became ataxic and convulsed before death had consumed a dead pigeon in the area in which poultry were dying from H5N1 [44]. Tigers from the large compound in Thailand had been fed cooked chicken carcasses or pork during the outbreak but had presumably been fed raw poultry carcasses approximately 12 days before the onset of clinical disease [48].

A large group of cats were housed in an animal shelter in Austria that also had a holding area of poultry [46]. A swan was brought to this shelter and died within 24 hours of arrival. The swan, along with 13 other birds, was identified as positive for H5N1 virus. The close proximity of the cats to the birds necessitated testing of cats for H5N1, and 3 of 40 tested positive. None of the positive cats exhibited any signs of respiratory distress or fever, however, and none had died by 50 days after initial exposure to the dead swan.

Experimental Disease

The severity of disease in wild and domestic cats prompted one group to experimentally infect domestic cats with HPAI H5N1 virus originally isolated from fatal disease in a human being [51,52]. Cats were exposed to H5N1 by intratracheal inoculation, by oral exposure through ingestion of virus-infected food, or by horizontal transmission in sentinel cats. All cats developed elevated body temperatures, decreased their activity levels, and had labored breathing. Six of the seven cats were euthanatized on day 7 of the experiment as part of a predetermined protocol. One cat died on day 6 of the experiment.

In one report documenting experimental infection in a small group of dogs, the results demonstrated viral excretion and seroconversion but no evidence of disease [53].

In the most recent study, Giese and colleagues [54], looked at transmissibility of an HPAI H5N1 virus, originally isolated from a cat, among dogs and cats. All the directly inoculated dogs developed mild pyrexia (39.2°–39.7°C) and conjunctivitis, but only three of four dogs were positive by RT-PCR and infectious virus was not recovered for any of the dogs. Uninfected contact cats remained clinically normal throughout the experiment, and none of the samples tested were positive by RT-PCR. Conversely, directly inoculated cats developed high fevers (>40°C), decreased activity, conjunctivitis, and labored breathing. Two of the cats were euthanatized 5 days after inoculation for humane reasons. None of the contact uninfected dogs developed symptoms, sera were negative for antibodies, and multiple samples were all negative by RT-PCR. Thus, it is unlikely that cats or dogs could serve as amplifying hosts or transmit the virus to contact human beings.

Gross and Histologic Pathology Findings

Pulmonary congestion, hemorrhage, and edema with variable severity of lung consolidation were the predominant gross lesions recorded for the cats that died of natural disease [43,44,46,48,49]. Additionally, numerous tissues were affected by multifocal hemorrhages involving the gastrointestinal tract and unspecified lymph nodes. Lesions in experimentally infected cats were primarily confined to the thoracic cavity, with varied proportions of lung being consolidated. The cats that were infected through ingestion of virus-infected chicks additionally had enlargement of and multifocal petechiation affecting the lymphoid structures of the head and neck.

Histologically, all the cats had evidence of bronchiolitis and alveolitis with neutrophilic and histiocytic bronchointerstitial pneumonia and pulmonary congestion and edema. Only the cats with natural disease had the severely hemorrhagic lesions affecting their lungs.

Two of the index large cats (one tiger and one leopard), the naturally diseased domestic cat, all the tigers necropsied from the second zoo outbreak, and all the cats experimentally infected with H5N1 (brains from the sentinel cats were not examined) had encephalitis, and most had evidence of leptomeningitis [43,44,48,51,52]. In nearly all cases, mononuclear cells infiltrated the perivascular space, and most had scattered variable gliosis. In a few cases, there were multifocal areas of necrosis within the neuropil complete with neutrophilic and macrophagic infiltration and variable neuronal necrosis.

In most cases reported, immunohistochemical stains for influenza A detected antigen within the nucleus or cytoplasm of neurons in the brain in addition to airway epithelial cells within the sections of lung.

Diagnosis

Unfortunately, cats that are febrile with respiratory distress could be afflicted with a multitude of pathogens. With the addition of depression and ataxia, one would have to include avian influenza as a possible cause for these symptoms. The index of suspicion should increase if birds are dying in the area. Blood can be collected to determine the presence of antibodies to HPAI H5N1 virus using various commercial available products. Swab samples from the respiratory tract or rectum can be assessed by RT-PCR for the presence of viral genomic nucleotides using primers specific for the H, N, or nucleocapsid genes [55].

Prevention and Control

The evidence of exposure to infected birds and the experimental evidence of infection after ingestion of virus-infected poultry confirm that cats are at risk in areas in which poultry and other birds are dying from H5N1 virus. Yet, the actual number of dogs and cats that succumbed to HPAI was extremely low. Cats that develop encephalitic disease are unlikely to respond to supportive therapy. Thus, minimizing exposure of cats to possible sources of infection is the best means of prevention.

BORNA DISEASE VIRUS

Borna disease (BD) is a sporadic progressive neurologic disease that primarily affects horses and sheep [56]. It received its name from the city of Borna in Saxony, Germany, where many horses died as the result of an epidemic of neurologic disease in the late 1800s. Much later, in the 1920s, it would be recognized that a virus caused the disease. BD virus is now known to infect a wider variety of species in a wider geographic range, and the first reports of BD causing disease in cats first appeared in the mid-1970s, when Kronevi first described a neurologic disease in cats in Sweden [57]. Since that original report, BD virus has been better characterized in the cat and there are rare reports of BD in dogs [57–63].

BD virus is a neurotropic pathogen of the new family Bornaviridae that causes sporadic progressive polioencephalomyelitis. Known to cause disease primarily in horses and sheep, it has been reported much less frequently in dogs and cats [56]. Specific regions of Germany were initially considered endemic for this disease, but it has since been confirmed as a pathogen in multiple other regions, including Switzerland, Japan, Austria, and Belgium, and confirmed based on serologic evidence in the Netherlands, France, Iran, Poland, and North America [56]. Its genome has been well characterized, and the putative nucleoprotein, designated p40, and putative phosphoprotein, designated p24, are exploited as molecular markers of infection [56]. Some researchers believe that BD virus may be associated with certain neuropsychiatric diseases in human beings, and thus may be a zoonotic pathogen, but opinions vary widely [64].

Surveillance Data for Dogs and Cats

Initial studies in Sweden determined that in cats with evidence of neurologic clinical symptoms compatible with BD, 44% (11 of 24) were serologically positive for BDV [57]. Additional surveys have been performed and the percentages positive range from a low of 3.3% (1 of 30) of cats in Finland to a high of 42.5% (3480) of cats in Turkey with antibodies to BDV [65–67]. One study noted that cats concurrently serologically positive for feline immunodeficiency virus (FIV) were more likely to be positive for BDV virus in cats tested in Germany [67]. In a Japanese study, 66.7% (10 of 15) of cats with neurologic disorders had antibodies in their sera to p24 or p40 [60]. Serologic surveys have not been documented in dogs.

Natural Disease

BD is believed to be the cause of a syndrome referred to as "staggering disease" in cats [57]. The clinical syndrome is characterized by hind-limb ataxia, drastic behavioral changes, lumbosacral pain, and an inability to retract claws in a small percentage of cases. Less commonly, cats become hypersensitive to sound and light, have impaired vision, and develop seizures.

Two reports exist that characterize neurologic disease in dogs associated with BD virus [62,63]. In one case, a 2-year-old husky dog from Austria became anorexic and lethargic and then developed severe CNS signs despite therapy, but those signs are not further characterized [62]. This dog was humanely euthanatized. In the second case, a 3-year-old Welsh corgi developed sudden hypoesthesia, tremors, and circling with hypersalivation. The dog became comatose and died.

Experimental Disease

Two strains of BD virus were used to study the pathogenesis of BD virus infection in cats: a rabbit-attenuated BD virus originally isolated from a horse and a recently isolated BD virus from a cat with staggering disease [59]. All cats were inoculated intracerebrally because the route of infection in natural disease remains undetermined. All the cats in this study seroconverted by the time the study was terminated regardless of the strain of virus used. Three of eight experimentally infected cats developed clinical disease. One cat became excessively shy by 20 days after infection, along with hind-limb ataxia and repetitive circling. These signs normalized by 27 days after infection, however. The remaining two cats developed hind-limb ataxia by 2.5 months after infection. Necropsy examinations confirmed meningoencephalitis of varying degrees in all three cats.

Gross and Histologic Pathology Findings

Cats that have been experimentally inoculated or naturally infected have similar histologic lesions that differ based on regions of the brain affected [58,59]. Lesions include nonsuppurative inflammation infiltrating the perivascular space comprising primarily lymphocytes, histiocytes, and occasional plasma cells. Nodules comprising lymphocytes and macrophages are scattered primarily in the gray matter and can be associated with neuronal degeneration and neuronal necrosis. The brain stem is most severely affected. Meningitis is seen throughout the entire CNS tissue examined. In natural infections, the olfactory bulb, medulla of the cerebellum, and brain stem are most severely affected. In experimental infections, the frontal cortex, basal nuclei, and rostral brain stem are most severely affected. Differences may simply be a reflection of variation of inoculation methods. Inclusion bodies have not been reported in natural or experimental infections in cats.

In dogs, a nonsuppurative meningoencephalitis is characterized by perivascular infiltrates by lymphocytes, histiocytes, and plasma cells. Neural necrosis and focal gliosis, along with endothelial swelling, were most severe in the rostral neocortex and pyriform lobes of the brain [62]. Neuronal satellitosis was also seen in the frontal neocortex [63]. Only in the Austrian dog were single or multiple characteristic intracytoplasmic and intranuclear eosinophilic viral inclusion bodies, also known as Joest-Degen inclusion bodies, identified in neurons [62].

Diagnosis
BD virus is confirmed by a wide variety of methods. BD virus–specific antibodies have been identified in sera and cerebrospinal fluid (CSF) using Western blot assays and ELISA assays. In addition to monoclonal antibodies, in situ hybridization and RT-PCR have been used on formalin-fixed tissues to identify BD viral antigen. A variety of culture techniques have been reported, but rabbit or rat embryonic brain cell lines are effective when virus isolation is used. Intracerebral inoculations of rabbits predictably results in disease in 3 to 4 weeks [56].

Prevention and Control
Unfortunately, this is a sporadic disease with no known or confirmed reservoir. For years, researchers have suspected rodents, but this has not yet been confirmed [56]. Thankfully, it is believed that most animals infected in the wild do not succumb to fatal disease. The zoonotic potential of this pathogen remains uncertain. There is limited evidence of reduced neuropsychiatric symptoms in patients with RNA from BDV detected in their circulating monocytic cells to the antiviral drug amantadine sulfate [64]. This same medication may be useful as a therapeutic agent in the future in dogs and cats. Currently, an effective vaccine is not available.

ENCEPHALITIC VIRUSES OF UNDETERMINED CLINICAL SIGNIFICANCE IN DOGS AND CATS
Other viruses have been reported to infect or result in disease, but none fit the criteria of being an emerging viral pathogen that causes disease. In one report, a few viruses were identified using IHC stains specific for certain viral antigens [14]. In this retrospective survey, brain sections from 53 dogs and 33 cats that had previously been diagnosed with nonsuppurative meningoencephalitis of unknown origin were subjected to a battery of IHC stains. The clinical signs were described for the entire group of animals based solely on information provided on the original necropsy submission forms, however. In 1 dog, there was a positive reaction to porcine herpesvirus I. Four dogs and 4 cats had detectable antigen for encephalomyocarditis virus. All the samples tested negative for BD virus, tick-borne encephalitis virus, feline leukemia virus, canine and feline herpesvirus, rabies virus, and CDV.

Another recent serologic survey determined that Florida dogs outside of the geographic region in which Everglades virus is normally detected in human and mosquito populations were serologically positive for this virus [68]. None of the dogs became sick as a result of being infected, however. These investigators speculate on the utility of dogs as a sentinel for human infection.

SUMMARY

Few viral pathogens resulting in encephalitis in dogs and cats have emerged over the past decade or so. All are the result of penetration through presumed species barriers and all are considered zoonoses or possible zoonotic pathogens. In all cases, encephalitis is a rare event that has low morbidity but high mortality. More viruses are likely to emerge as pathogenic in our domesticated carnivorous companions as our habitats continue to overlap with the shrinking wildlife habitats. Hopefully, however, none reach the level of distinction that was once held by rabies virus.

References

[1] Wilkinson L. History. In: Jackson AC, Wunner WH, editors. Rabies. 2nd edition. Amsterdam: Academic Press; 2007. p. 1–21.

[2] Smithburn KC, Hughes TP, Burke AW, et al. A neurotropic virus isolated from the blood of a native of Uganda. American Journal of Tropical Medicine 1940;20:471–92.

[3] Brinton MA. The molecular biology of West Nile virus: a new invader of the Western Hemisphere. Annu Rev Microbiol 2002;56:371–402.

[4] Komar N, Panella NA, Boyce E. Exposure of domestic mammals to West Nile virus during an outbreak of human encephalitis, New York City, 1999. Emerg Infect Dis 2001;7(4):736–8.

[5] Lancotti RS, Roehrig JT, Deubel V, et al. Origin of the West Nile virus responsible for an outbreak of encephalitis in the northeastern United States. Science 1999;286(5448):2333–7.

[6] Bin H, Grossman Z, Pokamunski S, et al. West Nile fever in Israel 1999–2000 from geese to humans. Ann N Y Acad Sci 2001;951(Dec):127–42.

[7] Komar N. West Nile virus: epidemiology and ecology in North America. Adv Virus Res 2004;61:185–234.

[8] Burt FJ, Grobbelaar AA, Leman PA, et al. Phylogenetic relationships of southern African West Nile virus isolates. Emerg Infect Dis 2002;8(8):820–6.

[9] Simpson VR, Kuebard G. A fatal case of Wesselsbron disease in a dog. Vet Rec 1979;105(4):329.

[10] Lichtensteiger CA, Heinz-Taheny K, Osborne TA, et al. West Nile virus encephalitis and myocarditis in wolf and dog. Emerg Infect Dis 2003;9(10):1303–6.

[11] Buckweitz S, Kleiboeker S, Marioni K, et al. Serological, reverse transcriptase-polymerase chain reaction, and immunohistochemical detection of West Nile virus in a clinically affected dog. J Vet Diagn Invest 2003;15(4):324–9.

[12] Read RW, Rodrigue DB, Summers BA. West Nile virus encephalitis in a dog. Vet Pathol 2005;42(2):219–22.

[13] Cannon AB, Luff JA, Brault AC, et al. Acute encephalitis, polyarthritis, and myocarditis associated with West Nile virus infection in a dog. J Vet Intern Med 2006;20:1219–23.

[14] Schwab S, Herden C, Seeliger F, et al. Non-suppurative meningoencephalitis of unknown origin in cats and dogs: an immunohistochemical study. J Comp Pathol 2007;136:96–110.

[15] Komar N. West Nile viral encephalitis. Rev Sci Tech 2000;19:166–76.

[16] Botha EM, Markotter W, Wolfaardt M, et al. Genetic determinants of virulence in pathogenic lineage 2 West Nile virus strains. Emerg Infect Dis 2008;14(2):222–30.

[17] Anonymous. Update: West Nile virus activity—eastern United States, 2000. MMWR Morb Mortal Wkly Rep 2000;49(46):1044–7.

[18] Kramer LD, Bernard KA. West Nile virus in the Western Hemisphere. Curr Opin Infect Dis 2001;14:519–25.

[19] Lindsey NP, Kuhn S, Campbell GL, et al. West Nile virus neuroinvasive disease incidence in the United States, 2002–2006. Vector -Borne Zoonotic Dis 2008;8:35–9.

[20] Available at: http://www.phac-aspc.gc.ca/wnv-vwn/nsr-rns_e.html. Accessed March 10, 2008.

[21] Blackburn NK, Reyers F, Berry WL, et al. Susceptibility of dogs to West Nile virus: a survey and pathogenicity trial. J Comp Pathol 1989;100:59–66.
[22] Kile JC, Panella NA, Komar N, et al. Serologic survey of cats and dogs during an epidemic of West Nile virus infection in humans. J Am Vet Med Assoc 2005;226(8): 1349–53.
[23] Ozkul A, Yildirim Y, Pinar D, et al. Serological evidence of West Nile virus (WNV) in mammalian species in Turkey. Epidemiol Infect 2006;134:826–9.
[24] Karaca K, Bowen RA, Austgen LE, et al. Recombinant canarypox vectored West Nile virus (WNV) vaccine protects dogs and cats against a mosquito WNV challenge. Vaccine 2005;23:3808–13.
[25] Austgen LE, Bowen RA, Bunning ML, et al. Experimental infection of cats and dogs with West Nile virus. Emerg Infect Dis 2004;10(1):82–6.
[26] Bowen RA, Rouge MM, Siger L, et al. Pathogenesis of West Nile virus infection in dogs treated with glucocorticoids. Am J Trop Med Hyg 2006;74(4):670–3.
[27] Eaton BT, Border CC, Middleton D, et al. Hendra and Nipah viruses: different and dangerous. Nat Rev Mircobiol 2006;4(1):23–35.
[28] Murray K, Rogers R, Selvey L, et al. A novel Morbillivirus pneumonia of horses and its transmission to humans. Emerg Infect Dis 1995;1(1):31–3.
[29] Murray K, Selleck P, Hooper P, et al. A morbillivirus that caused fatal disease in horses and humans. Science 1995;268(5207):94–7.
[30] Westbury HA. Hendra virus disease in horses. Rev Sci Tech 2000;19(1):151–9.
[31] Chua KB, Bellini WJ, Rota A, et al. Nipah virus: a recently emergent deadly paramyxovirus. Science 2000;288(5470):1432–5.
[32] Westbury HA, Hooper PT, Selleck PW, et al. Equine Morbillivirus pneumonia: susceptibility of laboratory animals to the virus. Aust Vet J 1995;72(7):278–9.
[33] Parashar UD, Sunn LM, Ong F, et al. Case-control study of risk factors for human infection with a new zoonotic paramyxovirus, Nipah virus, during a 1998–1999 outbreak of severe encephalitis in Malaysia. J Infect Dis 2000;181(5):1755–9.
[34] Epstein JH, Rahman SA, Zambriski JA, et al. Feral cats and risk for Nipah virus transmission. Emerg Infect Dis 2006;12(7):1178–9.
[35] Hooper P, Zaki S, Daniels P, et al. Comparative pathology of the diseases caused by Hendra and Nipah viruses. Microbes Infect 2001;3(4):315–22.
[36] Hooper PT, Westbury HA, Russell GM. The lesions of experimental equine morbillivirus disease in cats and guinea pigs. Vet Pathol 1997;34:323–9.
[37] Anonymous. Update: outbreak of Nipah virus—Malaysia and Singapore, 1999. MMWR Morb Mortal Wkly Rep 1999;48(16):335–7.
[38] Westbury HA, Hooper PT, Brouwer SL, et al. Susceptibility of cats to equine Morbillivirus. Aust Vet J 1996;74(2):132–4.
[39] Middleton DJ, Westbury HA, Morrissy CJ, et al. Experimental Nipah virus infection in pigs and cats. J Comp Pathol 2002;126:124–36.
[40] Claas ECJ, de Jong JC, van Beek R, et al. Human influenza virus A/HongKong/156/97 (H5N1) infection. Vaccine 1998;16(9/10):977–8.
[41] Li KS, Guan Y, Smith GJD, et al. Genesis of a highly pathogenic and potentially pandemic H5N1 influenza virus in eastern Asia. Nature 2004;430:209–13.
[42] Horimoto T, Kawaoka Y. Pandemic threat posed by avian influenza A viruses. Clin Microbiol Rev 2001;14(1):129–49.
[43] Keawchareon J, Oraveerakul K, Kuiken T, et al. Avian influenza H5N1 in tigers and leopards. Emerg Infect Dis 2004;10(12):2189–91.
[44] Songserm T, Amonsin A, Jam-on R, et al. Avian influenza H5N1 in naturally infected domestic cat. Emerg Infect Dis 2006;12(4):681–3.
[45] Butler D. Thai dogs carry bird-flu virus, but will they spread it? Nature 2006;439:773.
[46] Leschnik M, Weikel J, Mostl K, et al. Subclinical infection with avian influenza A (H5N1) virus in cats. Emerg Infect Dis 2007;13(2):243–7.

[47] Paltrinieri S, Spagnolo V, Giordano A, et al. Influenza virus type A serosurvey in cats. Emerg Infect Dis 2007;13(4):662–4.

[48] Thanawongnuwech R, Amonsin A, Tantilertcharoen R, et al. Probable tiger-to-tiger transmission of avian influenza H5N1. Emerg Infect Dis 2005;11(5):699–701.

[49] Klopfleisch R, Wolf PU, Uhl W, et al. Distribution of lesions and antigen of highly pathogenic avian influenza virus A/Swan/Germany/R65/06 (H5N1) in domestic cats after presumptive infection by wild birds. Vet Pathol 2007;44(3):261–8.

[50] Songserm T, Amonsin A, Jam-on R, et al. Fatal avian influenza A H5N1 in a dog. Emerg Infect Dis 2006;12(11):1744–7.

[51] Kuiken T, Rimmelzwaan G, van Riel D, et al. Avian H5N1 influenza in cats. Science 2004;306:241.

[52] Rimmelzwaan GF, van Riel D, Baars M, et al. Influenza A virus (H5N1) infection in cats causes systemic disease with potential novel routes of virus spread within and between hosts. Am J Pathol 2006;168(1):176–83.

[53] Maas R, Tacken M, Ruuls L, et al. Avian influenza (H5N1) susceptibility and receptors in dogs. Emerg Infect Dis 2007;13(8):1219–21.

[54] Giese M, Harder TC, Teifke JP, et al. Experimental infection and natural contact exposure of dogs with avian influenza virus (H5N1). Emerg Infect Dis 2008;14(2):308–10.

[55] Thiry E, Zicola A, Addie D, et al. Highly pathogenic avian influenza H5N1 virus in cats and other carnivores. Vet Microbiol 2007;122:25–31.

[56] Rott R, Herzog S, Richt JA. Borna disease. In: Coetzer JAW, Tustin RC, editors. 2nd edition, Infectious diseases of livestock, vol. 2. Oxford (Oxfordshire): Oxford University Press; 2004. p. 1368–72.

[57] Lundgren A-L, Ludwig H. Clinically diseased cats with non-suppurative meningoencephalomyelitis have Borna disease virus-specific antibodies. Acta Vet Scand 1993;34:101–3.

[58] Lundgren A-L. Feline non-suppurative meningoencephalomyelitis. A clinical and pathological study. J Comp Pathol 1992;107:411–25.

[59] Lundgren A-L, Johannisson A, Zimmermann W, et al. Neurological disease and encephalitis in cats experimentally infected with Borna disease virus. Acta Neuropathol 1997;93(3): 391–401.

[60] Nakamura Y, Watanabe M, Kamitani W, et al. High prevalence of Borna disease virus in domestic cats with neurologic disorders in Japan. Vet Microbiol 1999;70:153–69.

[61] Kamhieh S, Flower RLP. Borna disease virus (BDV) infection in cats. A concise review based on current knowledge. Vet Q 2006;28(2):65–73.

[62] Weissenböck H, Nowotny N, Caplazi P, et al. Borna disease in a dog with lethal meningoencephalitis. J Clin Microbiol 1998;36(7):2127–30.

[63] Okamoto M, Kagawa Y, Kamitani W, et al. Borna disease in a dog in Japan. J Comp Pathol 2002;126:312–7.

[64] Bode L, Ludwig H. Borna disease virus infection, a human mental-health risk. Clin Microbiol Rev 2003;16(3):534–45.

[65] Helps CR, Turan N, Bilal D, et al. Detection of antibodies to Borna disease virus in Turkish cats by using recombinant p40. Vet Rec 2001;149:647–50.

[66] Kinnunen PM, Billich C, Ek-Kommonen C, et al. Serological evidence for Borna disease virus infection in humans, wild rodents, and other vertebrates in Finland. J Clin Virol 2007;38: 64–9.

[67] Huebner J, Bode L, Ludwig H. Borna disease virus infection in FIV-positive cats in Germany. Vet Rec 2001;149:152.

[68] Coffey LL, Crawford C, Dee J, et al. Serologic evidence of widespread Everglades virus activity in dogs, Florida. Emerg Infect Dis 2006;12(12):1873–9.

Vet Clin Small Anim 38 (2008) 879–901

VETERINARY CLINICS
SMALL ANIMAL PRACTICE

ELSEVIER
SAUNDERS

Retroviral Infections of Small Animals

Stephen P. Dunham, BVSc, PhD, CertSAC, MRCVS[a],*,
Elizabeth Graham, MVB, MVM, PhD, MRCVS[b]

[a]Division of Veterinary Infection and Immunity, Institute of Comparative Medicine,
University of Glasgow, Faculty of Veterinary Medicine, Bearsden Road, Glasgow, G61 1QH, UK
[b]Division of Pathological Sciences, Institute of Comparative Medicine,
University of Glasgow, Faculty of Veterinary Medicine, Bearsden Road, Glasgow, G61 1QH, UK

Retroviral infections of the domestic cat are common. Representatives of three viral genera frequently infect cats: *Lentivirinae*, *γ-Retroviridae*, and *Spumavirinae*. Feline leukemia virus (FeLV), a γ-retrovirus, and feline immunodeficiency virus (FIV), a lentivirus, are pathogenic viruses that are transmitted exogenously (from cat to cat). Feline foamy virus (a spumavirus), although transmissible, is considered nonpathogenic [1], with a recent study showing no association between the presence of antibodies to the virus and clinical disease [2]. In addition, the genome of all domestic cats contains genetic elements derived from ancient retroviral infections of their ancestors, so-called "endogenous retroviruses," which are not transmitted exogenously between cats but are passed vertically by means of the germ line [3]. In contrast, there are no well-characterized retroviral infections of dogs, although there have been periodic reports of the isolation of retrovirus-like particles from dogs with clinical disease that could be compatible with retroviral infection [4–7].

RETROVIRUS GENOME

The basic genome structure of the family of retroviruses is similar. Virions contain two copies of single-stranded RNA with *gag*, *pol*, and *env* genes. These encode the core proteins of the virus (*gag*), enzymes responsible for virus replication (*pol*), and surface proteins (*env*). In addition, lentiviruses, such as FIV and spumaviruses, encode other accessory proteins that enable the virus to regulate their life cycle more tightly or productively infect a broader range of cell types (Fig. 1).

Retroviruses, like most RNA viruses, are subject to a large degree of genetic variation. This may arise by two major mechanisms. Mutation may occur because of the inability of the virus replicative enzymes to "proof read" during replication. Secondly, recombination can occur between similar genomes or parts of genomes. The genetic variation for FIV is greater than that seen for

*Corresponding author. *E-mail address*: s.dunham@vet.gla.ac.uk (S.P. Dunham).

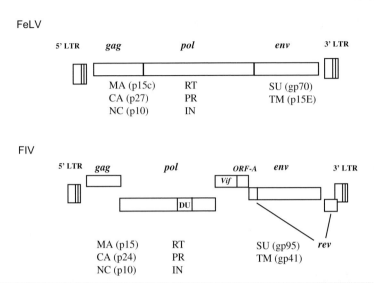

Fig. 1. Genomic structure of FeLV and FIV proviruses. The major genes are *gag* (group specific antigen), *pol* (polymerase), and *env* (envelope). The major viral proteins shown are as follows: MA, matrix; CA, capsid; NC, nucleocapsid; RT, reverse transcriptase; PR, protease; IN, integrase; SU, surface protein; and TM, transmembrane protein. FIV also has several accessory genes, including *rev*, *vif*, DU (dUTPase), and ORF-A (open reading frame A). LTR, long terminal repeat regions that flank the integrated provirus and regulate gene expression.

FeLV. Presumably, greater changes in FeLV render the virus less viable than FIV. FIV exists in at least five subtypes or clades, A to E, which are defined based on their *env* sequence; there may be up to 30% divergence between samples from different clades [8,9]. Different clades predominate in different geographic regions; for example, clade A viruses are common in northern Europe and the western United States, whereas clade B viruses predominate in southern Europe and the eastern United States [8,10].

FeLV subtypes are classified as FeLV-A, FeLV-B, and FeLV-C, based on their *env* sequence. FeLV-A is the predominant subtype that is isolated from all infected cats and is transmitted exogenously between animals. FeLV-B arises in approximately 50% of cats because of recombination between FeLV-A and endogenous FeLV-related retroviruses in the cat genome. Infection with FeLV-B viruses may influence the course of disease; for example, infection can accelerate the generation of lymphomas or increase virus neuropathogenicity [3]. FeLV-C viruses arise rarely in cats infected with FeLV-A because of point mutations in the *env* gene and invariably cause the rapid development of fatal anemia. FeLV-B and FeLV-C viruses are usually not transmissible to other cats. Rather, such viruses arise de novo as a chance event in some cats infected with FeLV-A. More recently, a variant of FeLV associated with severe immunodeficiency has been described. This variant, designated FeLV-T, has a marked tropism for T lymphocytes [11,12]. FeLV-T is most closely related to FeLV-A, from which it evolves during infection as a result of multiple mutations throughout the *env* gene.

RETROVIRUS LIFE CYCLE

An overview of the retrovirus life cycle is shown in Fig. 2. This typical retroviral life cycle has several consequences that have an impact on the host-virus relation. First, the process of copying RNA to DNA by reverse transcription is not completely accurate, such that errors are introduced into the viral genome. As outlined previously, this leads to genetic variation in subsequent progeny virions. Although some of these may be defective, a number may have altered antigenicity, and thus have a survival advantage, enabling them to evade the developing host immune response. Second, the process of integration leads to persistence of the viral genome in the cell. If the virus remains inactive, producing no viral proteins or progeny virions, it remains largely invisible to the host immune system—so-called "latent infection."

CELLULAR RECEPTORS FOR FELINE RETROVIRUSES

During the past decade, our knowledge of the cellular receptors used by FIV and FeLV has increased dramatically. FIV, like HIV, requires primary and

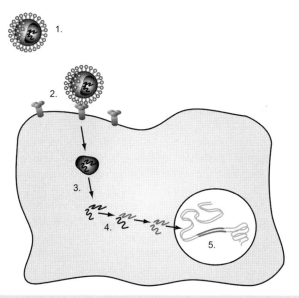

Fig. 2. Simplified overview of retrovirus life cycle. 1. Virus particle. 2. Virus binds to cellular receptors by means of its envelope surface proteins (Env) and subsequently enters the cell after fusion with the cell membrane. 3. Viral RNA genome is released from the viral core. 4. RNA genome is copied by the viral enzyme "reverse transcriptase" into a DNA copy (cDNA), and this DNA is then duplicated to produce double-stranded DNA, which then enters the cell nucleus. 5. Viral DNA is spliced into the host genome by the viral integrase protein, where it resides for the life of the host cell as provirus.

secondary receptors. The primary receptor is CD134, expressed on feline CD4$^+$ T lymphocytes, B lymphocytes, and activated macrophages [13,14]. The secondary receptor CXCR4, a chemokine receptor, is analogous to that used by HIV; this receptor alone is sufficient for infection with some laboratory isolates of FIV. FeLV targets cells through interaction with several receptors, determined by the virus subtype [15]. FeLV-B uses the sodium-dependant inorganic phosphate transporters Pit1 and Pit2 [12,16]. FeLV-C uses a trans- porter molecule present on hemopoietic cells as described elsewhere in this article [17,18]. Recently, the receptor for FeLV-A has been characterized as a putative thiamine transport protein [19]. The marked T-lymphocyte tropism of FeLV-T is attributable to the alteration in the receptor used by the virus to enter cells. FeLV-T uses a coreceptor (FeLIX) expressed on T lymphocytes. Curiously, this receptor sequence is identical to that of a truncated endogenous FeLV envelope. Improvements in understanding retroviral receptor use help to explain the pathogenesis of these viral infections and allow for the possible development of therapies directed at blocking virus-receptor interactions.

FELINE RETROVIRUSES AND DISEASE
Feline retroviruses are perhaps the most important cause of infectious disease in domestic cats. FeLV and FIV cause a spectrum of diseases with a degree of overlap, such that their differentiation is rarely possible on clinical grounds alone (Table 1). Despite these similarities, the nature of infection with each virus and the subsequent immune response and pathogenesis are quite differ- ent. Importantly, recovery from FIV infection has never been documented, although most cats exposed to FeLV are able to clear their infection.

FELINE IMMUNODEFICIENCY VIRUS INFECTION AND DISEASE
FIV was first reported in 1986, when it was isolated from sick cats in a cattery in California. The animals showed clinical signs that included anorexia, leukope- nia, pyrexia, gingivitis, diarrhea, and weight loss [20]. Since then, FIV has been reported throughout the world, with a prevalence of up to 28% in some countries, and has become an important disease of pet cats [21]. Most FIV infec- tions occur after a bite wound from an infected cat, presumably through the inoculation of virus or virus-infected cells [22]. FIV thus more commonly affects free-ranging intact male cats, which are more likely to be involved in fights. Transmission of FIV from a queen to her kittens may also occur after experimen- tal infection, with evidence of virus transmission in utero, during parturition, or postpartum by means of infected colostrum or milk [23–26]. Transmission of infection by such routes in naturally infected cats seems to be less common. Unlike HIV, neither oronasal nor venereal spread has been documented for FIV.

The course of FIV infection, like HIV, can be classified into several stages (Fig. 3). After virus entry, lymphoid and myelomonocytic cells become infected, with virus integration into the host genome leading to persistent infec- tion. FIV replicates rapidly within dendritic cells, macrophages, and CD4$^+$ T lymphocytes, leading to the release of new virus particles, and a peak viremia

Table 1
Diseases caused by feline retroviruses

	FeLV	FIV	Feline spumavirus
Virus genus	γ-Retrovirus	Lentivirus	Spumavirus
Outcome of infection	Approximately 60% of cats develop protective immunity; 30% of cats become persistently viremic and develop FeLV-related disease, typically within 3 years	All animals become persistently infected; transient disease coincides with initial period of viremia; thereafter, animals remain ostensibly healthy for many years; increased viremia in latter stages of disease is associated with opportunistic infections	Virus is thought to be nonpathogenic
Disease spectrum	Lymphomas Leukemia Anemia Enteritis Immunosuppression Abortion and infertility	Immunosuppression Chronic persistent infections B-cell lymphomas Leukemia Neurologic disease Anemia	None recognized

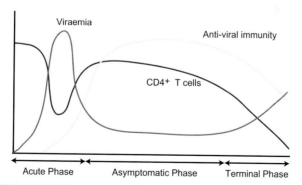

Fig. 3. Time course of infection with FIV. The acute phase of infection lasts up to several months with an initial peak in plasma viremia and a decrease in CD4⁺ T lymphocytes. With the development of antiviral immunity, the plasma viral load decreases and CD4⁺ lymphocyte counts largely recover. During the asymptomatic phase, which may last many years, plasma viral loads remain relatively low, but a slow decline in CD4⁺ lymphocyte counts can be seen. In the terminal stages of infection, the antiviral immune response wanes and plasma viral loads again increase. During this stage, a marked immunodeficiency results in secondary bacterial and opportunistic infections.

occurs 8 to 12 weeks after infection. During this acute phase of infection, mild to moderate clinical signs associated with the initial uninhibited growth of the virus, such as anorexia, depression, and pyrexia, may be observed [27]. These conditions generally subside rapidly, although signs like generalized lymphade-nopathy, attributable to increased number and size of active follicular germinal centers, may continue for several weeks or months. Virus replication is gener-ally brought under control by the developing immune response to the virus. $CD8^+$ FIV-specific cytotoxic T lymphocytes (CTLs) can be detected in the blood within 1 week of infection [28]. Later in the course of infection, at around the same time as the peak in virus load, anti-FIV antibodies, including virus neutralizing antibodies (VNAs), appear in the plasma [29]. A decrease in plasma viral load associated with virus-specific immune responses heralds the beginning of the "asymptomatic" phase, which can last for many years and, in many cases, for the life of the cat; during this time, the cat is quite healthy.

The final outcome of FIV infection is variable. It is becoming increasingly clear, however, that FIV infection does not necessarily result in life-threatening disease. During the asymptomatic phase, the plasma viral load is stable but a progressive decline in $CD4^+$ T-lymphocyte numbers occurs. Functional assays also show a reduced ability of T lymphocytes to respond effectively to antigen or mitogen [9]. In some animals, this decline may be sufficient to re-sult in a functional immunodeficiency that leads to opportunistic infections causing clinical disease and death. In the later stages of disease, sometimes re-ferred to as "AIDS-related complex," secondary bacterial infections are com-mon, particularly of the upper respiratory tract, oral cavity, and conjunctivae. Other clinical diseases include chronic enteritis, skin disease, neu-rologic disorders, and neoplasia. Should the infected cat survive beyond this stage, a clinical picture similar to AIDS in HIV-infected patients may be seen, with the development of opportunist infections, such as those caused by poxvirus, *Cryptococcus*, *Mycobacteria*, *Demodex*, and other parasites. In contrast to the severity of such terminal stages of the disease, one study of a closed household of 26 cats observed only slow spread of FIV between animals over a 10-year period, and it did not seem to cause any significant disease [30]. The outcome of infection may be determined, at least in part, by the vir-ulence of the infecting virus, but it is likely that multiple factors are responsible (eg, concurrent disease, genetic factors leading to resistance or susceptibility).

FELINE LEUKEMIA VIRUS INFECTION AND DISEASE

Over 40 years since its discovery in 1964, FeLV remains an important disease of domestic cats. Most FeLV infections occur after oronasal spread of the virus in saliva from viremic cats [31,32]. Such transmission is favored in multicat households, in which mutual grooming and sharing of food and water bowls is common. Viral replication initially occurs in the oropharynx, particularly tonsillar lymphocytes and macrophages. Thereafter, virus spread occurs to draining lymph nodes and blood. After the development of viremia, FeLV is able to spread rapidly to its preferred target tissues: those containing rapidly dividing lymphoid, myeloid, and epithelial cells [33]. This phase of infection is critical. If the developing immune response is able to contain the virus, infection may be extinguished. Approximately 60% of cats exposed to FeLV recover, in that infectious virus cannot be isolated from their blood. In approximately 30% of infected cats, the virus load exceeds the ability of the immune response to eliminate infection and the animals develop a persistent viremia. The relative proportion of animals that recover or develop persistent infection is affected by several factors, including the age of the animal at the time of exposure, virus dose, route of exposure, and concurrent disease. Most persistently infected cats subsequently develop FeLV-related disease and die within 3 years of infection. FeLV-related diseases include neoplasia, such as lymphomas and leukemia, and non-neoplastic diseases, such as anemia, enteritis, and secondary infections attributable to immunosuppression.

It is not yet clear whether the immune response can eliminate FeLV proviral DNA from recovered cats that are no longer antigenemic or viremic. Some investigators have consistently detected FeLV provirus in recovered cats [34–36], whereas other laboratories have reported a provirus-negative status in some cats after recovery [37]. Once provirus has integrated into the hematopoietic stem cells, total elimination of infection seems improbable, because progeny cells also carry proviral DNA. The clinical significance of provirus-positive aviremic cats is uncertain; however, it is likely that viral replication does not resume in most of these cats.

Feline Leukemia Virus and Tumor Development

FeLV is a simple retrovirus, bearing only the genes necessary for replication, and as such, the virus lacks specific cancer-causing oncogenes. Nonetheless, at its peak, FeLV was responsible for most tumors of hematopoietic origin in the cat, accounting for one third of all feline tumors in the United States. [33,38]. The virus is thought to promote tumor development in two major ways. First, insertional mutagenesis, in which the sequences in the provirus that usually drive virus replication lead to activation of cellular oncogenes [39]. The second mechanism is termed *transduction*, in which an FeLV provirus acquires cellular oncogenes, such as *myc*, by recombination [40–42]. Such recombinant viruses can lead to rapid tumor development [43].

Feline Leukemia Virus–Associated Lymphoma

The most common FeLV-associated tumor is lymphoma, a malignant tumor of lymphocytes [33]. Lymphoma may originate within any organ and spread to other sites is classified according to the primary site of involvement: mediastinal (thymic), alimentary, multicentric, or extranodal [44]. Extranodal lymphoma originates from a single site other than the alimentary tract or thymus, such as the skin, eyes, kidneys, or nervous system. FeLV-associated lymphoma tends to be T lymphocyte in origin, whereas nonretroviral lymphoma is derived from B or T lymphocytes [43]. Historically, multicentric lymphoma was the most common form identified in the United States [43], whereas in Scotland, alimentary lymphoma was most common form [45,46]. It is not known whether this accurately reflects a geographic variation in distribution or whether other laboratory-based factors, such as the use of different diagnostic protocols, could account for the difference [47]. What is clear, however, is that different forms of lymphoma are variably associated with FeLV viremia and age. Three-quarters of thymic lymphoma cases are associated with FeLV (FeLV antigenemic or viremic cats), and most occur in young cats [33], whereas alimentary lymphoma cases are more prevalent in older cats. A much lower percentage of alimentary lymphoma, approximately 25%, is associated with FeLV [48]. Ninety percent of multicentric lymphoma cases are associated with FeLV, and these tend to occur in cats aged approximately 4 years.

The declining prevalence of FeLV infection, attributable largely to effective test and elimination programs, has been accompanied by a decreasing number of FeLV-associated lymphoma cases. Data from the 1970s illustrated that up to 70% of lymphoma cases were FeLV-antigenemic or FeLV-viremic [43]. More recently, only 14.5% of lymphoma cases examined at a US institute (1983–2003) were retrovirus associated (FIV-positive or FeLV-positive), with more than 50% of retrovirus-positive cases diagnosed before 1991 [49]. In this study, the most common form of lymphoma was alimentary (53.9%), with mediastinal lymphomas being relatively uncommon (5.7%). A possible genetic predisposition among the Siamese breed to mediastinal lymphoma has been proposed, however [49].

The classification of lymphomas as FeLV-negative based solely on the absence of antigenemia or viremia probably underestimates the prevalence of tumors associated with FeLV. FeLV proviral DNA sequences have been detected in a proportion of lymphoma tissues from nonantigenemic cats [50–53] as well as in nonlymphoma tissues, typically bone marrow cells [43,54]. In one study, nonantigenemic cats in which provirus was detected in tumor tissue by polymerase chain reaction (PCR), showed a higher proportion of non–B and non–T-cell tumors and fewer B cell tumors compared with provirus-negative or nonantigenemic cats [52]. The provirus-positive or nonantigenemic cats had a median age of 10 years, which is significantly older than viremic cats with lymphoma. Such studies suggest that the immune response in some animals may have been sufficient to contain virus replication but not to prevent the later development of lymphoid tumors.

Feline Leukemia Virus–Associated Anemia

The incidence of anemia is high among FeLV-viremic cats [55]. Weakly regenerative anemia secondary to concurrent FeLV disease, such as lymphoma, myeloproliferative disease, or immunosuppressive disease, is common. In addition, more than half of cats with lymphoma may develop anemia in the absence of bone marrow infiltration, possibly because of hemolysis [55]. Primary nonregenerative anemia is an important but rare syndrome in viremic cats associated with FeLV-C [55,56]. Initial studies revealed that FeLV-C greatly impairs the differentiation of early erythroid progenitor cells within the bone marrow, inhibiting erythrocyte production [57,58]. More recent work has established that the receptor for FeLV-C (FLVCR1) is a heme-exporting protein [17,18]. Binding of FeLV-C to its receptor culminates in a fatal accumulation of heme in the erythroid progenitor cells [59], accounting for the specific loss of the erythrocyte series.

Other Feline Leukemia Virus–Associated Diseases

FeLV has a predilection for rapidly dividing intestinal crypt cells. FeLV-associated enteritis is a non-neoplastic condition associated with persistent FeLV infection, characterized by diarrhea, hematemesis, and anemia [43]. Viral proteins can be detected immunohistochemically in the small intestines of FeLV-positive cats, particularly gp70 and p15E [60]. A variety of reproductive abnormalities have also been associated with FeLV. Abortion, fetal resorption, infertility, stillbirths, and neonatal deaths are reported to occur in more than 80% of FeLV-positive cats [48]. Rarely, FeLV has been associated with skin disease in the form of giant-cell dermatosis or the formation of epidermal footpad horns [53,61].

FELINE LEUKEMIA VIRUS IMMUNOLOGY

The immune mechanisms that influence outcome after exposure to FeLV have yet to be fully resolved. Virus-neutralizing antibodies (VNAs) have been detected in peripheral blood from FeLV-exposed cats and can confer protection in some circumstances [62]. Recently, the role of CTLs in mediating vaccinal protection and recovery has been investigated [63,64].

Virus-Neutralizing Antibodies

VNAs predominantly target epitopes located on the FeLV envelope and trans-membrane proteins gp70 and p15E [65–67]. Neonatal kittens born to FeLV-immune queens may be protected by passively transferred maternal antibodies [62], and VNAs are often present at higher levels in recovered cats. Nonetheless, VNAs do not necessarily mediate recovery from infection. In a recent longitudinal FeLV immunopathogenesis study, all cats that recovered from experimental challenge developed significant VNA titers. The appearance of VNAs followed, or was concurrent with, clearance of infectious virus, however [68]. Similar findings have been reported in other studies [65,69,70]. Moreover, VNAs may be present in the serum of cats that later become persistently viremic [70]. Nonetheless, most recovered cats produce higher VNA titers, which peak earlier, than persistently viremic cats [70,71]. The presence of a high VNA titer is therefore a good indicator of protective immunity in a naturally exposed cat. It seems that the Feline Virus Unit at the University of Glasgow is the only laboratory currently offering this test.

Cell-Mediated Immune Response

The ability of CTLs to control FeLV replication and mediate recovery has been defined. Cats that recover after experimental exposure to FeLV develop early virus-specific CTL responses, which are maintained until infectious virus is cleared from the blood [68]. Cats that fail to recover from FeLV infection after experimental challenge show delayed and short-lived virus-specific CTLs. In addition, the adoptive transfer of a single infusion of mixed virus-specific $CD4^+$ and $CD8^+$ T lymphocytes was shown to reduce the proviral DNA burdens in persistently infected cats, indicating a direct role for virus-specific T lymphocytes in the control of FeLV viremia [68].

Virus-specific CTLs are also important in protective vaccinal immunity. High levels of FeLV-specific CTLs are present in blood and lymphoid tissues from FeLV DNA-vaccinated protected cats [47,63]. Virus-specific CTLs occur at higher levels in vaccinated protected and unvaccinated recovered cats compared with unvaccinated persistently viremic cats.

Immunosuppression

More cats die from immunosuppression than from lymphoma or any other FeLV-associated disease [43]. In vitro studies have demonstrated functional suppression of T and B lymphocytes from persistently FeLV-infected kittens, although T lymphocytes were more profoundly affected [72–76]. Humoral immune responses to T-lymphocyte–dependent antigens were weaker in infected cats, prompting suggestions that an early $CD4^+$ T-lymphocyte malfunction in the persistently viremic cats might adversely affect the humoral response [77]. This hypothesis was supported by the observation that B-lymphocyte numbers markedly declined in the early stages of illness but later resolved [76].

The immunosuppressive effect of FeLV does not seem to be restricted to B and T lymphocytes. Persistently viremic cats are highly susceptible to opportunistic bacterial and fungal infections, which might indicate impaired innate immunity. Indeed, polymorphonuclear (PMN) cells from FeLV-infected cats were shown to be functionally impaired in vitro [78].

Evidence exists to suggest that the FeLV transmembrane protein p15E may be partly responsible for the immunosuppressive effects of FeLV [79]. Purified p15E suppressed PMN activity and human and feline mitogenic and antigenic responses [73,80,81]. FeLV seems to act directly to exert a general but temporary impairment on the ability of the T lymphocyte to produce, and respond to, certain cytokines [82–84]; in one study, this seemed to be mediated by p15E.

DIAGNOSIS OF FELINE LEUKEMIA VIRUS AND FELINE IMMUNODEFICIENCY VIRUS INFECTION
Diagnosis of Feline Leukemia Virus Infection
Many assays have been developed to detect FeLV infection. Diagnostic tests are available to detect the FeLV p27 capsid protein, whole virus, or integrated proviral DNA. An understanding of the type of test used, and the viral component measured, is critical to allow correct interpretation of an FeLV test result.

Screening tests, such as commercial immunochromatography tests and laboratory ELISAs, detect free FeLV p27 protein in plasma. With the prevalence of FeLV in the United Kingdom now decreasing to 1.4% among the healthy cat population [85], a high positive predictive value (PPV; the proportion of positive test cats in a population that are correctly diagnosed by a test) is extremely important. A recent study comparing several commercial immunochromatography products available showed a large variability in test sensitivity and specificity [86]. The study was based on data from US cats, and PPV values ranging from 62% to 90% were calculated [86]. A low PPV score leads to a high proportion of false-positive results, emphasizing the need for confirmation of all positive results attained through screening.

Several tests are available to confirm positive screening tests: virus isolation, immunofluorescence, and PCR. Virus isolation detects the presence of whole infectious virions; positive results therefore indicate active viremia. Detection of viremia is of critical importance in the control of FeLV infection and in the diagnosis of FeLV-related disease, because viremic cats are infectious to other cats and most persistently viremic cats succumb to an FeLV-related disease within 3 years. The assay may require prolonged culture times of up to 10 days, however, and few diagnostic laboratories now have the expertise to conduct this test. Immunofluorescence assays detect the presence of FeLV p27 within circulating leukocytes on a fixed blood smear, and therefore accurately detect the viremic state [87]. These assays can thus be used as a more rapid alternative to virus isolation. Virus isolation and immunofluorescence tests are considered the "gold standards" for FeLV diagnosis. PCR is a specific and sensitive assay used to detect FeLV proviral DNA in circulating leukocytes. It is likely that all cats exposed to FeLV become provirus-positive and remain so, however, even after recovery [35]. Quantitative PCR assays can correlate high virus loads with viremia, but, ultimately, PCR assays cannot distinguish between viremic and nonviremic cats. Such a distinction is crucial to the effective control of FeLV infection and to the diagnosis of FeLV-related disease.

Positive p27 antigenemia does not always correlate with viremia [88]. Such a discordant state is likely to reflect early recovery or early infection and occurs in as many as 10% of positive antigen results. Cats giving discordant results should be retested in 4 to 12 weeks when the test results usually concur. Rarely, discordant test results can be attributable to the intermittent release of the p27 protein by a small local or sequestered infection [89]; these cats may give discordant results for years. Such cats are potentially infectious to other cats, and their viral status should be monitored closely.

Latently infected cats are characterized by being neither antigenemic nor viremic; however, infectious virus can be isolated from the bone marrow of these cats after a short period of in vitro culture. Virus isolation from bone marrow remains the only method to detect latently infected cats definitively [36,90]. Latently infected cats have an increased incidence of FeLV-related disease compared with uninfected cats [91]. Most latently infected cats eliminate virus within 30 months of exposure [92].

Cats can be tested for FeLV infection at any age; kittens should be tested twice from birth at 12-week intervals. Viremia can be transient; thus, if clinical signs are absent or mild, viremic cats should be retested in 12 to 16 weeks. If still viremic, this is likely indicative of persistent viremia.

Diagnosis of Feline Immunodeficiency Virus Infection

Because FIV infection correlates with the presence of high anti-FIV antibody titers, most commercially available FIV screening tests detect specific anti-FIV antibodies. The prevalence of FIV is higher than that of FeLV in the United Kingdom and in the United States, resulting in higher PPV scores for FIV commercial screening tests [86]. Some of the commercial screening tests available apparently show 100% sensitivity to FIV, indicating that all positive cats are detected using this method, provided that the test is used correctly. No test is 100% specific, however, creating the possibility of false-positive results. To avoid this, all positive results obtained from a commercial kit should be confirmed using another test method.

Western blot tests, immunofluorescence assays, virus isolation, and PCR assays are all used as confirmatory tests for FIV infection. Western blot tests and immunofluorescence assays detect anti-FIV antibodies, and Western blot analysis is considered the gold standard for the diagnosis of FIV infection. Recent difficulties in distinguishing between antibodies associated with vaccination and antibodies generated as a result of natural infection [93] have focused attention on methods available to detect virus rather than antibody. Virus isolation detects circulating infectious virus but is not widely available, because the assay is time-consuming to perform and requires considerable expertise. Many PCR assays have been designed to detect FIV viral or proviral DNA. Problems with poor sensitivity and specificity of commercial PCR assays seem to be widespread, however [94]. False-negative results can occur with PCR testing if viral loads are lower than the threshold of detection or if the primers have not been designed to recognize all FIV variants [95]. One alternative could be to use multiple antigens in an ELISA format. Kusuhara and colleagues [96], using such an approach, showed that it was possible to distinguish vaccinated from infected cats with an accuracy of 97% to 98%. Clearly, in the face of increasing use of FIV vaccination in pet cats, there is a need for improved methods to diagnose FIV infection.

When screening kittens for FIV, the FIV status of the queen should be considered. Maternal FIV-specific antibodies are transferred to all kittens in colostrum, potentially giving rise to false-positive results when using antibody-based tests [97]. If the queen is FIV-positive or of unknown status, any FIV-positive kittens younger than the age of 16 weeks should be retested for anti-FIV antibodies once they have reached 16 weeks of age. It can also take up to 12 weeks for antibodies to develop after exposure to FIV; therefore, if contact with a known infected cat has occurred, testing should be performed 12 weeks after exposure.

VACCINATION AGAINST FELINE RETROVIRAL DISEASE

The development of successful vaccines against FeLV and, more recently, against FIV owes much to the dedicated efforts of several research groups worldwide. Many early attempts at developing FeLV and FIV vaccines were discouraging. The first experimental FeLV vaccines, which were based on live tumor cells, although effective, were shown to cause neoplasia in some vaccinated animals. Unfortunately, inactivated vaccines based on the same cells showed poor efficacy. Despite these early setbacks, further research efforts led to licensing of the first FeLV vaccine in 1985. Since that time, several improved vaccines have been developed. More recently, FIV vaccine development has endured similar setbacks. The first licensed FIV vaccine was released in 2002, however, a breakthrough that paves the way for future FIV vaccines.

Feline Leukemia Virus Vaccination

There are currently five types of FeLV vaccines licensed for use in the United Kingdom. A similar range of products is available in the United States. These include: whole inactivated virions, inactivated gp70 and feline oncornavirus cell membrane antigens (FOCMAs) prepared from FeLV-infected tissue culture cells, recombinant envelope protein (p45), and, more recently, a live canarypox recombinant vaccine that expresses Gag, Env, and protease proteins. All vaccines, with the exception of the canarypox vaccine, contain adjuvant.

Efficacy and Safety of Feline Leukemia Virus Vaccines

The efficacy and safety of FeLV vaccines continue to be questioned. Ideally, an effective vaccine should protect FeLV-exposed cats from viremia and latent infection and confer no lasting harmful effect. In experimental trials, however, no vaccine fully protects cats against the development of persistent and latent infection [98,99]. In terms of safety, FeLV vaccines have been linked with the development of feline injection site sarcomas (FISSs), which are particularly aggressive and frequently fatal [100].

The introduction of FeLV vaccination coincided with a decrease in the prevalence of FeLV. This is unlikely to be attributable to vaccination alone. The widely used "test and remove" policy has had a considerable impact on disease prevalence [101]. The efficacy of the vaccines has been difficult to establish in the field because of the low prevalence of the disease, the natural phenomenon of age-related immunity, and the difficulties presented in establishing and evaluating the correlates of protection. Furthermore, few independent vaccine efficacy studies are available. Many such studies have been conducted or supported by the manufacturer, and results are often conflicting [99]. To date, no vaccine has successfully managed to prevent transient viremia when evaluated in a controlled study [99], or even consistently to protect against the development of persistent viremia [99]. In a more recent study, neither of two vaccines under test prevented minimal virus replication and provirus integration after experimental challenge [35]. It is not clear whether it is possible to achieve sterilizing immunity after vaccination, with conflicting data arising from different laboratories [35,36,102,103]. Indeed, it may well be that limited virus replication is required to elicit protective immunity [35,104]. The mechanism of protection conferred by commercially available vaccines has not been investigated. VNAs are unlikely to be the main component of protective immunity after vaccination, because significant VNA titers are not observed using some vaccine preparations until after challenge [35,105,106].

Furthermore, in a recent FeLV DNA experimental vaccine study [47], protection was conferred without eliciting anti-FeLV VNAs. Indeed, infectious virus was cleared from the blood before virus-specific VNAs were generated after challenge, indicating that VNAs were not involved in recovery. Virus-specific CTLs are likely to be important in protective vaccinal immunity. In recent experimental vaccine studies, high levels of FeLV-specific CTLs were present in blood and lymphoid tissues from FeLV DNA-vaccinated protected cats [47,63].

Safety concerns center on the development of FISSs in some FeLV-vaccinated cats. These tumors are believed to evolve from chronic granulomatous inflammatory changes induced by trauma in tumor-susceptible cats [107]. In the early stages, vaccines were causally implicated for several reasons. First, the localization was suggestive, with 84% located between the shoulder blades [108], and, second, many vaccines induce a strong local inflammatory reaction [100]. In 2003, a multi-institutional prospective trial was undertaken to clarify the association between vaccine brand and the development of feline sarcomas [108]. This trial failed to identify a particular vaccine brand or manufacturer at fault, however, and the researchers considered that vaccination was unlikely to be the sole cause of FISSs [108]. Regarding the continued use of feline vaccine products, the European Union–appointed Committee for Veterinary Medicinal Products (CVMP) suggested a case-by-case risk assessment but did not promote the recommendations made by the US-based Vaccine-Associated Feline Sarcoma Task Force, advocating different vaccination sites for each vaccine [100]. The American Association of Feline Practitioners (AAFP) has also recommended that vaccination protocols should be based on the circumstances of individual cats, such that only cats at risk for contracting disease should be vaccinated. Overall, the incidence of FISS is relatively low and stable: 0.63 sarcomas per 10,000 cats in the United States [109].

Despite the ongoing concerns regarding vaccine efficacy and safety, it must be remembered that the most important role of vaccination is the prevention of persistent viremia and the development of FeLV-associated fatal disease. Even if currently available vaccines are unable to provide sterilizing immunity, all provide significant protection against persistent viremia and contribute to significant reductions in proviral and viral loads [35].

Feline Leukemia Virus Vaccine Development

The search for more effective vaccines has prompted experimentation with novel adjuvants [110], live viral vectors [111], and DNA vaccination [47]. Experimental DNA vaccines have been developed for many infectious diseases with some early successes [112–114]. Their efficacy in clinical trials has been disappointing, however [115]. The coadministration of biologic adjuvants in the form of cytokines, chemokines, or costimulatory molecules may enhance the immune response elicited by DNA vaccines [116–118]. Using such an approach, an experimental FeLV DNA vaccine containing *gag*, *pol*, and *env* genes, adjuvanted with interleukin (IL)-12 and IL-18 cytokine DNA, was able to prevent the development of persistent and transient viremia [47]. A follow-up study demonstrated that IL-18 was the most important cytokine adjuvant in the vaccine; of six animals vaccinated with the FeLV DNA vaccine and IL-18 plasmid alone, all were protected against viremia and five of six were protected against latent infection [119].

Feline Immunodeficiency Virus Vaccination

In comparison to vaccination for FeLV, the development of a vaccine for FIV has been particularly difficult. This is largely because of the nature of the lentiviral infection and its ability to evade and sabotage the host immune response. Clearly, the parallels with HIV are marked [120]. A large number of experimental FIV vaccines have been tested, including conventional inactivated virus and infected cell vaccines and more modern approaches based on DNA vaccination or bacterial vectors (for detailed reviews, the reader is referred to other articles Refs. [121–123]). These have shown variable success; however, in general, complete protection has been difficult to achieve. Despite the associated difficulties, an FIV vaccine based on inactivated virus–infected cells was first licensed in the United States in 2002 [121] and has subsequently become available in several other countries, including Canada, Australia, and New Zealand.

The licensed vaccine (Fel-O-Vax FIV; Fort Dodge, Overland Park, Kansas) is made from a feline cell line infected with two subtypes of FIV. This inactivated vaccine is able to provide improved protection in experimental trials, compared with a single subtype vaccine, against challenge with several different viral strains [124–126]. Protection does not extend to all virus isolates, however [127]. Thus, although the current vaccine represents a step forward, there remains the need for an improved vaccine. In particular, as already mentioned, the widespread use of an FIV vaccine that contains whole inactivated virus also raises a problem for diagnosis of FIV infection because it induces an antibody response indistinguishable from that induced by viral infection.

FUTURE DEVELOPMENTS IN SMALL ANIMAL RETROVIROLOGY

Retrovirus Evolution

The potential for retroviruses to mutate in their host raises the possibility that new subtypes may arise in the future, particularly for FIV, with its large potential for genetic variation. This may have an impact on the ability of any prophylactic vaccines to protect against infection if new emerging viruses are able to escape the specific immune response induced by vaccination. It is also possible that they may be associated with atypical disease. The precedent for this has been established for FIV, in which a variant clade B virus has recently been described in a group of feral cats in Texas. The virus, FIV-TX53, may be more pathogenic than prevalent clade B viruses [128,129].

Treatment of Feline Immunodeficiency Virus– and Feline Leukemia Virus–Infected Cats

As our understanding of the mechanisms of retroviral infection increases, so do the opportunities to develop new therapies tailored for FIV and FeLV. Potential new treatments include the use of specific receptor antagonists that block the binding of the virus envelope to host cell receptors and fusion inhibitors that prevent the subsequent fusion of virus and cellular membranes; such drugs have been the focus of much research and development for HIV therapy [130]. Other stages of the retrovirus life cycle, including nuclear entry [131], integration [132], and virus assembly [133], are also prime targets for drug therapy. An alternative approach is the targeting of the glycan groups present on the surface of the viral envelope glycoproteins; such an approach is able to block HIV infection in vitro. A second benefit of this novel treatment may be to direct virus mutation to lose some of these glycan moieties that normally shield the virus from the binding of antiviral antibodies, rendering the virus more amenable to neutralization [134]. Unfortunately, most of these treatments are unlikely to become available for small animal treatment because they are likely to be highly specific for HIV, have significant research and development costs, and may be associated with unexpected side effects in nonhuman species. Recent improvements in our understanding of the mechanisms of FIV and FeLV viral entry may, however, pave the way for development of drugs that block viral entry.

RNA interference (RNAi) is a technology that has generated great excitement as a potential for modifying cellular gene expression, including that of exogenous viruses (for reviews, the reader is referred to other articles Refs. [135,136]). Because the technology only requires knowledge of the sequence of target genes (eg, FeLV or FIV sequences), it is readily transferable to small animals. FeLV, in particular, is an attractive target, in view of the lack of alternative therapies and its relatively conserved sequence.

A large number of experimental treatments have been used in an attempt to clear or reduce the viremia associated with persistent FeLV infection. These include passive transfer of antiviral antibody and use of biologic response modifiers, including cytokines, antiretroviral drugs, and bone marrow transplantation. In most cases, these treatments have, at best, resulted in some clinical improvement, but the long-term reversal of viremia is extremely rare. Similar treatments have been unsuccessful in the control of FIV-associated viremia. Unlike the treatment of HIV, the use of antiretroviral drugs in cats has met with limited success, and they have been associated with significant toxicity, precluding long-term treatment [137,138].

In the absence of specific antiviral agents, current therapy for FeLV and FIV-infected cats relies on the appropriate treatment of any associated clinical disease. Supportive therapy therefore includes treatment of secondary infections, chemotherapy for lymphoma and other neoplasms, prophylactic use of vaccines against common feline infectious disease, and prevention of parasitic disease. In any case, it is important to consider the isolation of an infected cat so that it does not act as a source of infection for healthy animals.

Canine Retroviruses

The lack of characterized retroviruses in dogs is perhaps surprising. However, there have been sporadic reports of the detection of retroviral particles or retroviral activity in cells derived from dogs with immunosuppression [5], cutaneous T-cell lymphoma [7], large granular lymphocytic leukemia [6], and myeloproliferative disease [4]. The lack of further cases may be attributable to inadequate investigation or may accurately reflect a low incidence of such infections in the dog. Nevertheless, with the increased availability and sophistication of molecular methods for studying viral infections, further studies are warranted to ascertain their true incidence.

SUMMARY

FIV and FeLV remain important infections of domestic cats. Eradication programs for FeLV, based on test and removal schemes and vaccination, have significantly reduced the incidence of the disease. However, the prognosis for a persistently infected cat remains poor. FIV infections remain common, and the impact of a recently released vaccine has yet to be documented. Development of improved vaccines would be welcome for both diseases, especially FIV. In the meantime, there is an urgent need for reliable methods for diagnosis of FIV in the face of vaccination. It is possible that the future may also bring novel treatments that may offer some hope to cats that succumb to persistent infection with FeLV or FIV. Unfortunately, it is unlikely that drugs developed for treating human retroviral disease are going to be suitable for treatment of infected cats.

References

[1] Jarrett O. Strategies of retrovirus survival in the cat. Vet Microbiol 1999;69(1–2):99–107.
[2] Romen F, Pawlita M, Sehr P, et al. Antibodies against Gag are diagnostic markers for feline foamy virus infections while Env and Bet reactivity is undetectable in a substantial fraction of infected cats. Virology 2006;345(2):502–8.
[3] Roy-Burman P. Endogenous env elements: partners in generation of pathogenic feline leukemia viruses. Virus Genes 1995;11(2–3):147–61.
[4] Sykes GP, King JM, Cooper BC. Retrovirus-like particles associated with myeloproliferative disease in the dog. J Comp Pathol 1985;95(4):559–64.
[5] Modiano JF, Getzy DM, Akol KG, et al. Retrovirus-like activity in an immunosuppressed dog: pathological and immunological findings. J Comp Pathol 1995;112(2):165–83.
[6] Ghernati I, Corbin A, Chabanne L, et al. Canine large granular lymphocyte leukemia and its derived cell line produce infectious retroviral particles. Vet Pathol 2000;37(4):310–7.
[7] Ghernati I, Auger C, Chabanne L, et al. Characterization of a canine long-term T cell line (DLC 01) established from a dog with Sézary syndrome and producing retroviral particles. Leukemia 1999;13(8):1281–90.
[8] Sodora DL, Shpaer EG, Kitchell BE, et al. Identification of three feline immunodeficiency virus (FIV) env gene subtypes and comparison of the FIV and human immunodeficiency virus type 1 evolutionary patterns. J Virol 1994;68(4):2230–8.
[9] Burkhard MJ, Dean GA. Transmission and immunopathogenesis of FIV in cats as a model for HIV. Curr HIV Res 2003;1(1):15–29.
[10] Bachmann MH, Mathiason-Dubard C, Learn GH, et al. Genetic diversity of feline immunodeficiency virus: dual infection, recombination, and distinct evolutionary rates among envelope sequence clades. J Virol 1997;71(6):4241–53.
[11] Anderson MM, Lauring AS, Burns CC, et al. Identification of a cellular cofactor required for infection by feline leukemia virus. Science 2000;287(5459):1828–30.

[12] Anderson MM, Lauring AS, Robertson S, et al. Feline Pit2 functions as a receptor for subgroup B feline leukemia viruses. J Virol 2001;75(22):10563–72.

[13] Willett BJ, McMonagle EL, Logan N, et al. Probing the interaction between feline immunodeficiency virus and CD134 by using the novel monoclonal antibody 7D6 and the CD134 (Ox40) ligand. J Virol 2007;81(18):9665–79.

[14] Shimojima M, Miyazawa T, Ikeda Y, et al. Use of CD134 as a primary receptor by the feline immunodeficiency virus. Science 2004;303(5661):1192–5.

[15] Willett BJ, Hosie MJ, Neil JC, et al. Common mechanism of infection by lentiviruses. Nature 1997;385(6617):587.

[16] Takeuchi Y, Vile RG, Simpson G, et al. Feline leukemia virus subgroup B uses the same cell surface receptor as gibbon ape leukemia virus. J Virol 1992;66(2):1219–22.

[17] Quigley JG, Burns CC, Anderson MM, et al. Cloning of the cellular receptor for feline leukemia virus subgroup C (FeLV-C), a retrovirus that induces red cell aplasia. Blood 2000;95(3):1093–9.

[18] Tailor CS, Willett BJ, Kabat D. A putative cell surface receptor for anemia-inducing feline leukemia virus subgroup C is a member of a transporter superfamily. J Virol 1999;73(8):6500–5.

[19] Mendoza R, Anderson MM, Overbaugh J. A putative thiamine transport protein is a receptor for feline leukemia virus subgroup A. J Virol 2006;80(7):3378–85.

[20] Pedersen NC. Virologic and immunologic aspects of feline infectious peritonitis virus infection. Adv Exp Med Biol 1987;218:529–50.

[21] Ishida T, Washizu T, Toriyabe K, et al. Feline immunodeficiency virus infection in cats of Japan. J Am Vet Med Assoc 1989;194(2):221–5.

[22] Yamamoto JK, Hansen H, Ho EW, et al. Epidemiologic and clinical aspects of feline immunodeficiency virus infection in cats from the continental United States and Canada and possible mode of transmission. J Am Vet Med Assoc 1989;194(2):213–20.

[23] O'Neil LL, Burkhard MJ, Hoover EA. Frequent perinatal transmission of feline immunodeficiency virus by chronically infected cats. J Virol 1996;70(5):2894–901.

[24] O'Neil LL, Burkhard MJ, Diehl LJ, et al. Vertical transmission of feline immunodeficiency virus. AIDS Res Hum Retroviruses 1995;11(1):171–82.

[25] Sellon RK, Jordan HL, Kennedy-Stoskopf S, et al. Feline immunodeficiency virus can be experimentally transmitted via milk during acute maternal infection. J Virol 1994;68(5):3380–5.

[26] Allison RW, Hoover EA. Feline immunodeficiency virus is concentrated in milk early in lactation. AIDS Res Hum Retroviruses 2003;19(3):245–53.

[27] Callanan JJ, Thompson H, Toth SR, et al. Clinical and pathological findings in feline immunodeficiency virus experimental infection. Vet Immunol Immunopathol 1992;35(1–2):3–13.

[28] Beatty JA, Willett BJ, Gault EA, et al. A longitudinal study of feline immunodeficiency virus-specific cytotoxic T lymphocytes in experimentally infected cats, using antigen-specific induction. J Virol 1996;70(9):6199–206.

[29] Fevereiro M, Roneker C, Laufs A, et al. Characterization of two monoclonal antibodies against feline immunodeficiency virus gag gene products and their application in an assay to evaluate neutralizing antibody activity. J Gen Virol 1991;72(Pt 3):617–22.

[30] Addie DD, Dennis JM, Toth S, et al. Long-term impact on a closed household of pet cats of natural infection with feline coronavirus, feline leukaemia virus and feline immunodeficiency virus. Vet Rec 2000;146(15):419–24.

[31] Jarrett WF, Martin WB, Crighton GW, et al. Transmission experiments with leukemia (lymphosarcoma). Nature 1964;202:566–7.

[32] Jarrett WF, Crawford EM, Martin WB, et al. A virus-like particle associated with leukemia (lymphosarcoma). Nature 1964;202:567–9.

[33] Hardy WD. Haematopoietic tumours of cats. J Am Anim Hosp Assoc 1981;17:921–40.

[34] Hofmann-Lehmann R, Huder JB, Gruber S, et al. Feline leukaemia provirus load during the course of experimental infection and in naturally infected cats. J Gen Virol 2001;82:1589–96.

[35] Hofmann-Lehmann R, Tandon R, Boretti FS, et al. Reassessment of feline leukaemia virus (FeLV) vaccines with novel sensitive molecular assays. Vaccine 2006;24(8):1087–94.

[36] Hofmann-Lehmann R, Cattori V, Tandon R, et al. Vaccination against the feline leukaemia virus: outcome and response categories and long-term follow-up. Vaccine 2007;25(30): 5531–9.

[37] Tandon R, Cattori V, Gomes-Keller MA, et al. Quantitation of feline leukaemia virus viral and proviral loads by TaqMan(R) real-time polymerase chain reaction. J Virol Methods 2005;130(1–2):124–32.

[38] Dorn CR, Taylor DO, Schneider R, et al. Survey of animal neoplasms in Alameda and Contra Costa Counties, California. II. Cancer morbidity in dogs and cats from Alameda County. J Natl Cancer Inst 1968;40:307–18.

[39] Lenz J, Celander D, Crowther RL, et al. Determination of the leukaemogenicity of a murine retrovirus by sequences within the long terminal repeat. Nature 1984;308(5958): 467–70.

[40] Levy LS, Gardner MB, Casey JW. Isolation of a feline leukaemia provirus containing the oncogene *myc* from a feline lymphosarcoma. Nature 1984;308:853–6.

[41] Mullins JI, Brody DS, Binari RC, et al. Viral transduction of *c-myc* gene in naturally occurring feline leukaemias. Nature 1984;308:856–8.

[42] Neil JC, Hughes D, McFarlane R, et al. Transduction and rearrangement of the *myc* gene by feline leukaemia virus in naturally occurring T-cell leukaemias. Nature 1984;308: 814–20.

[43] Hardy WD. Feline oncoretroviruses. In: Levy JA, editor. The *Retroviridae*. New York: Plenum Press; 1993. p. 109–80.

[44] Guillermo Couto C. What is new on feline lymphoma? J Feline Med Surg 2001;3(4): 171–6.

[45] Crighton GW. The diagnosis of leukaemia in the cat. J Small Anim Pract 1969;10:571–7.

[46] Crighton GW. Lymphosarcoma in the cat. Vet Rec 1969;84:329–31.

[47] Hanlon L, Argyle D, Bain D, et al. Feline leukaemia virus DNA vaccine efficiency is enhanced by coadministration with interleukin-12 (IL-12) and IL-18 expression vectors. J Virol 2001;75(18):8424–33.

[48] Pedersen NC. Feline leukaemia virus infection. In: Pedersen NC, editor. Feline infectious diseases. Goleta (CA): American Veterinary Publications; 1988. p. 83–106.

[49] Louwerens M, London CA, Pedersen NC, et al. Feline lymphoma in the postfeline leukemia virus era. J Vet Intern Med 2005;19:329–35.

[50] Koshy R, Wong-Staal F, Gallo RC, et al. Distribution of feline leukaemia virus DNA sequences in tissues of normal and leukaemia domestic cats. Virology 1979;99:135–44.

[51] Koshy R, Gallo RC, Wong-Staal F. Characterization of the endogenous feline leukemia virus-related DNA sequences in cats and attempts to identify exogenous viral sequences in tissues of virus-negative leukemic animals. Virology 1980;103:434–45.

[52] Gabor LJ, Love DN, Malik R, et al. Feline immunodeficiency virus status of Australian cats with lymphosarcoma. Aust Vet J 2001;79(8):540–5.

[53] Favrot C, Wilhelm S, Grest P, et al. Two cases of FeLV-associated dermatoses. Vet Dermatol 2005;16:407–12.

[54] Hardy WD, McClelland AJ, Zuckerman EE, et al. Development of virus non-producer lymphosarcomas in pet cats exposed to FeLV. Nature 1980;288:90–2.

[55] Mackey L, Jarrett W, Jarrett O, et al. Anemia associated with feline leukaemia virus infection in cats. J Natl Cancer Inst 1975;54(1):209–17.

[56] Hoover EA, Kociba GJ, Hardy WD, et al. Erythroid hypoplasia in cats inoculated with feline leukaemia virus. J Natl Cancer Inst 1974;53(5):1271–6.

[57] Onions D, Jarrett O, Testa N, et al. Selective effect of feline leukaemia virus on early erythroid precursors. Nature 1982;296:156–8.

[58] Hoover EA, Mullins JI. Feline leukaemia virus infection and disease. J Am Vet Med Assoc 1991;199(10):1287–97.

[59] Quigley JG, Yang Z, Worthington MT, et al. Identification of a human heme exporter that is essential for erythropoiesis. Cell 2004;118(6):757–66.

[60] Kipar A, Kremendahl J, Grant CK, et al. Expression of viral proteins in feline leukaemia virus-associated enteritis. Vet Pathol 2000;37:129–36.

[61] Gross TL, Clark EG, Hargis AM, et al. Giant cell dermatosis in FeLV-positive cats. Vet Dermatol 1993;4(3):117–22.

[62] Jarrett O, Russell PH, Stewart MF. Protection of kittens from feline leukaemia virus infection by maternally-derived antibody. Vet Rec 1977;101:304–5.

[63] Flynn JN, Hanlon L, Jarrett O. Feline leukaemia viruses: protective immunity is mediated by virus-specific cytotoxic T lymphocytes. Immunology 2000;101:1–10.

[64] Flynn JN, Dunham SP, Mueller A, et al. Involvement of cytolytic and non-cytolytic T cells in the control of feline immunodeficiency virus infection. Vet Immunol Immunopathol 2002;85:159–70.

[65] Russell PH, Jarrett O. The occurrence of feline leukaemia virus neutralizing antibodies in cats. Int J Cancer 1978;22:351–7.

[66] Elder JH, McGee JS, Munson M, et al. Localization of neutralizing regions of the envelope gene of feline leukaemia virus by using anti-synthetic peptide antibodies. J Virol 1987;61: 8–15.

[67] Nick S, Klaws J, Friebel K, et al. Virus neutralizing and enhancing epitopes characterized by synthetic oligopeptides derived from the feline leukaemia virus glycoprotein sequence. J Gen Virol 1990;71:77–83.

[68] Flynn JN, Dunham SP, Watson V, et al. Longitudinal analysis of feline leukaemia virus-specific cytotoxic T lymphocytes: correlation with recovery from infection. J Virol 2002;76(5):2306–15.

[69] Hoover EA, Olsen RG, Hardy WD, et al. Feline leukaemia virus infection: age-related variation in response of cats to experimental infection. J Natl Cancer Inst 1976;57(2):365–9.

[70] Charreyre C, Pedersen NC. Study of feline leukaemia virus immunity. J Am Vet Med Assoc 1991;199(10):1316–24.

[71] Lutz H, Pedersen NC, Higgins J, et al. Humoral immune reactivity to feline leukaemia virus and associated antigens in cats naturally infected with feline leukaemia virus. Cancer Res 1980;40:3642–51.

[72] Hebebrand LC, Mathes LE, Olsen RG. Inhibition of concanavalin A stimulation of feline lymphocytes by inactivated feline leukaemia virus. Cancer Res 1977;37:4532–3.

[73] Hebebrand LC, Olsen RG, Mathes LE, et al. Inhibition of human lymphocyte mitogen and antigen response by a 15,000-dalton protein from feline leukaemia virus. Cancer Res 1979;39:443–7.

[74] Mathes LE, Olsen RG, Hebebrand LC, et al. Abrogation of lymphocyte blastogenesis by a feline leukaemia virus protein. Nature 1978;274:687–9.

[75] Perryman LE, Hoover EA, Yohn DS. Immunologic reactivity of the cat: immunosuppression in experimental feline leukaemia. J Natl Cancer Inst 1972;49:1357–65.

[76] Cockerell GL, Hoover EA, Krakowka S, et al. Lymphocyte mitogen reactivity and enumeration of circulating B- and T- cells during feline leukaemia virus infection in the cat. J Natl Cancer Inst 1976;57(5):1095–9.

[77] Trainin Z, Wernicke D, Ungar-Waron H, et al. Suppression of the humoral antibody response in natural antibody response in natural retrovirus infections. Science 1983;220: 858–9.

[78] Lafrado LJ, Olsen RG. Demonstration of depressed polymorphonuclear leukocyte function in nonviraemic FeLV-infected cats. Cancer Invest 1986;4(4):297–300.

[79] Copelan EA, Rinehart JJ, Lewis M, et al. The mechanism of retrovirus suppression of human T cell proliferation in vitro. J Immunol 1983;131(4):2017–20.

[80] Mathes LE, Olsen RG, Hebebrand LC, et al. Immunosuppressive properties of a virion polypeptide, a 15,000-dalton protein, from feline leukaemia virus. Cancer Res 1979;39:950–5.

[81] Lafrado LJ, Lewis MG, Mathes LE, et al. Suppression of in vitro neutrophil function by feline leukaemia virus (FeLV) and purified FeLV-p15E. J Gen Virol 1987;68:507–13.

[82] Orosz CG, Zinn NE, Olsen RG, et al. Retrovirus-mediated immunosuppression. II. FeLV-UV alters in vitro murine T lymphocyte behaviour by reversibly impairing lymphokine secretion. J Immunol 1985;135(1):583–90.

[83] Liu WT, Good RA, Trang LQ, et al. Remission of leukaemia and loss of feline leukaemia virus in cats injected with Staphylococcus protein A: association with increased circulating interferon and complement-dependent cytotoxic antibody. Proc Natl Acad Sci U S A 1984;81:6471–5.

[84] Engelman RW, Fulton RW, Good RA, et al. Suppression of gamma interferon production by inactivated feline leukaemia virus. Science 1984;227:1368–70.

[85] Muirden A. Prevalence of feline leukaemia virus and antibodies to feline immunodeficiency virus and feline coronavirus in stray cats sent to an RSPCA hospital. Vet Rec 2002;150(20): 621–5.

[86] Hartmann K, Griessmayr P, Schulz B, et al. Quality of different in-clinic test systems for feline immunodeficiency virus and feline leukaemia virus infection. J Feline Med Surg 2007;9(6): 439–45.

[87] Hardy WD, Old LJ, Hess PW, et al. Horizontal transmission of feline leukaemia virus. Nature 1973;244:266–9.

[88] Jarrett O. Overview of feline leukaemia virus research. J Am Vet Med Assoc 1991;199: 1279–81.

[89] Lutz H, Pedersen NC, Theilen GH. Course of feline leukemia virus infection and its detection by enzyme-linked immunosorbent assay and monoclonal antibodies. Am J Vet Res 1983;44(11):2054–9.

[90] Madewell BR, Jarrett O. Recovery of feline leukaemia virus from non-viraemic cats. Vet Rec 1983;112:339–42.

[91] Rojko JL, Hoover EA, Quackenbush SL, et al. Reactivation of latent feline leukaemia virus infection. Nature 1982;298:385–8.

[92] Pacitti AM, Jarrett O. Duration of the latent state in feline leukaemia virus infections. Vet Rec 1985;117:472–4.

[93] Levy JK, Crawford PC, Slater MR. Effect of vaccination against feline immunodeficiency virus on results of serologic testing in cats. J Am Vet Med Assoc 2004;225(10):1558–61.

[94] Bienzle D, Reggeti F, Wen X, et al. The variability of serological and molecular diagnosis of feline immunodeficiency virus infection. Can Vet J 2004;45(9):753–7.

[95] Steinrigl A, Klein D. Phylogenetic analysis of feline immunodeficiency virus in Central Europe: a prerequisite for vaccination and molecular diagnostics. J Gen Virol 2003;84(Pt 5):1301–7.

[96] Kusuhara H, Hohdatsu T, Seta T, et al. Serological differentiation of FIV-infected cats from dual-subtype feline immunodeficiency virus vaccine (Fel-O-Vax FIV) inoculated cats. Vet Microbiol 2007;120(3–4):217–25.

[97] MacDonald K, Levy JK, Tucker SJ, et al. Effects of passive transfer of immunity on results of diagnostic tests for antibodies against feline immunodeficiency virus in kittens born to vaccinated queens. J Am Vet Med Assoc 2004;225(10):1554–7.

[98] Jarrett O, Ganière J-P. Comparative studies of the efficacy of a recombinant feline leukaemia virus vaccine. Vet Rec 1996;138:7–11.

[99] Sparkes H. Feline leukaemia virus: a review of immunity and vaccination. J Small Anim Pract 1997;38:187–94.

[100] Kirpensteijn J. Feline injection site-associated sarcoma: is it a reason to critically evaluate our vaccination policies? Vet Microbiol 2006;117(1):59–65.

[101] Hardy WD, Hess PW, MacEwan G, et al. Biology of feline leukaemia virus in the natural environment. Cancer Res 1976;36:582–8.

[102] Torres AN, Mathiason CK, Hoover EA. Re-examination of feline leukemia virus: host relationships using real-time PCR. Virology 2005;332(1):272–83.

[103] Tandon R, Cattori V, Willi B, et al. Copy number polymorphism of endogenous feline leukemia virus-like sequences. Mol Cell Probes 2007;21(4):257–66.

[104] Klenerman P, Hengartner H, Zinkernagel RM. A non-retroviral RNA virus persists in DNA form. Nature 1997;390:298–301.

[105] Pedersen NC. Immunogenicity and efficacy of a commercial feline leukemia virus vaccine. J Vet Intern Med 1993;7:34–9.

[106] Hawks DM, Legendre AM, Rohrbach BW, et al. Antibody response of kittens after vaccination followed by exposure to feline leukaemia virus-infected cats. J Am Vet Med Assoc 1991;199(10):1463–9.

[107] Jelinek F. Postinflammatory sarcoma in cats. Exp Toxicol Pathol 2003;55:167–72.

[108] Kass PH, Spangler WL, Hendrick MJ, et al. Multicenter case-control study of risk factors associated with development of vaccine-associated sarcomas in cats. J Am Vet Med Assoc 2003;223(9):1283–92.

[109] Gobar GM, Kass PH. World Wide Web–based survey of vaccination practices, postvaccinal reactions, and vaccine site-associated sarcomas in cats. J Am Vet Med Assoc 2002;220(10):1477–82.

[110] Osterhaus A, Weijer K, Uytdehaag F, et al. Induction of protective immune response in cats by vaccination with feline leukemia virus iscom. J Immunol 1985;135:591–6.

[111] Willemse MJ, van Schooneveld SH, Chalmers WS, et al. Vaccination against feline leukaemia using a new feline herpesvirus type 1 vector. Vaccine 1996;14:1511–6.

[112] Boyer JD, Ugen KE, Chattergoon M, et al. DNA vaccination as anti-human immunodeficiency virus immunotherapy in infected chimpanzees. J Infect Dis 1997;176(6):1501–9.

[113] Fuller DH, Corb MM, Barnett S, et al. Enhancement of immunodeficiency virus-specific immune responses in DNA-immunized rhesus macaques. Vaccine 1997;15(8):924–6.

[114] Hosie MJ, Flynn JN, Rigby MA, et al. DNA vaccination affords significant protection against feline immunodeficiency virus infection without inducing detectable antiviral antibodies. J Virol 1998;72(9):7310–9.

[115] Donnelly JJ, Wahren B, Liu MA. DNA vaccines: progress and challenges. J Immunol 2005;175(2):633–9.

[116] Cohen A, Boyer JD, Weiner DB. Modulating the immune response to genetic immunization. FASEB J 1998;12(15):1611–26.

[117] Lee AH, Suk Suh Y, Chul Sung Y. DNA inoculations with HIV-1 recombinant genomes that express cytokine genes enhance HIV-1 specific immune responses. Vaccine 1999;17(5):473–9.

[118] Calarota SA, Weiner DB. Enhancement of human immunodeficiency virus type 1-DNA vaccine potency through incorporation of T-helper 1 molecular adjuvants. Immunol Rev 2004;199(1):84–99.

[119] O'Donovan LH, McMonagle EL, Taylor S, et al. A vector expressing feline mature IL-18 fused to IL-1[beta] antagonist protein signal sequence is an effective adjuvant to a DNA vaccine for feline leukaemia virus. Vaccine 2005;23(29):3814–23.

[120] Dunham SP. Lessons from the cat: development of vaccines against lentiviruses. Vet Immunol Immunopathol 2006;112(1–2):67–77.

[121] Uhl EW, Heaton-Jones TG, Pu R, et al. FIV vaccine development and its importance to veterinary and human medicine: a review FIV vaccine 2002 update and review. Vet Immunol Immunopathol 2002;90(3–4):113–32.

[122] Dunham SP, Jarrett O. FIV as a model for AIDS vaccine studies. In: Friedman H, Specter S, Bendinelli M, editors. In vivo models of HIV disease and control. New York: Springer; 2006. p. 293–332.

[123] Hosie MJ, Beatty JA. Vaccine protection against feline immunodeficiency virus: setting the challenge. Aust Vet J 2007;85(1–2):5–12.

[124] Pu R, Coleman J, Omori M, et al. Dual-subtype FIV vaccine protects cats against in vivo swarms of both homologous and heterologous subtype FIV isolates. AIDS 2001;15(10):1225–37.

[125] Kusuhara H, Hohdatsu T, Okumura M, et al. Dual-subtype vaccine (Fel-O-Vax FIV) protects cats against contact challenge with heterologous subtype B FIV infected cats. Vet Microbiol 2005;108(3–4):155–65.
[126] Pu R, Coleman J, Coisman J, et al. Dual-subtype FIV vaccine (Fel-O-Vax FIV) protection against a heterologous subtype B FIV isolate. J Feline Med Surg 2005;7(1):65–70.
[127] Dunham SP, Bruce J, MacKay S, et al. Limited efficacy of an inactivated feline immunodeficiency virus vaccine. Vet Rec 2006;158(16):561–2.
[128] Phadke AP, Concha-Bermejillo A, Wolf AM, et al. Pathogenesis of a Texas feline immunodeficiency virus isolate: an emerging subtype of clade B. Vet Microbiol 2006;115(1–3): 64–76.
[129] Weaver EA, Collisson EW, Slater M, et al. Phylogenetic analyses of Texas isolates indicate an evolving subtype of the clade B feline immunodeficiency viruses. J Virol 2004;78(4): 2158–63.
[130] Este JA, Telenti A. HIV entry inhibitors. Lancet 2007;370(9581):81–8.
[131] Suzuki Y, Craigie R. The road to chromatin-nuclear entry of retroviruses. Nat Rev Microbiol 2007;5(3):187–96.
[132] De Clercq E. HIV-chemotherapy and -prophylaxis: new drugs, leads and approaches. Int J Biochem Cell Biol 2004;36(9):1800–22.
[133] Brazil M. HIV-1. Viral assembly inhibitors on the horizon. Nat Rev Drug Discov 2005;4(9): 716–7.
[134] Balzarini J. Targeting the glycans of glycoproteins: a novel paradigm for antiviral therapy. Nat Rev Microbiol 2007;5(8):583–97.
[135] de Fougerolles A, Vornlocher HP, Maraganore J, et al. Interfering with disease: a progress report on siRNA-based therapeutics. Nat Rev Drug Discov 2007;6(6):443–53.
[136] Ketzinel-Gilad M, Shaul Y, Galun E. RNA interference for antiviral therapy. J Gene Med 2006;8(8):933–50.
[137] Hartmann K, Donath A, Beer B, et al. Use of two virustatica (AZT, PMEA) in the treatment of FIV and of FeLV seropositive cats with clinical symptoms. Vet Immunol Immunopathol 1992;35(1–2):167–75.
[138] Egberink HF, Hartman K, Horzinek MC. Chemotherapy of feline immunodeficiency virus infection. J Am Vet Med Assoc 1991;199(10):1485–7.

Vet Clin Small Anim 38 (2008) 903–917

VETERINARY CLINICS
SMALL ANIMAL PRACTICE

Vaccines for Emerging and Re-Emerging Viral Diseases of Companion Animals

David Scott McVey, DVM, PhD[a],*,
Melissa Kennedy, DVM, PhD[b]

[a]Nebraska Veterinary Diagnostic Center, Department of Veterinary and Biomedical Sciences,
College of Agriculture and Natural Resources, University of Nebraska-Lincoln,
PO Box 830907, Lincoln, NE 68583–0907, USA
[b]Department of Comparative Medicine, College of Veterinary Medicine, A205 Veterinary
Teaching Hospital, University of Tennessee, 2407 River Drive, Knoxville,
TN 37996–4543, USA

Vaccines for the prevention of viral diseases of companion animals have proved to be effective and safe. The risks and costs associated with use have generally been acceptable [1,2]. Nevertheless, there is a continuing and considerable investment to improve safety and efficacy profiles of vaccines in clinical use. A significant portion of the research and development investment is directed toward the development of efficacious vaccines for emerging or re-emerging diseases of companion animals. These infectious threats include new strains or mutant forms of old diseases (eg, rabies virus [RV], feline calicivirus [FCV]) or changes in the geographic distributions of diseases representing new threats to companion animal populations (RV and Lyssavirus [LV]). As the need to address immunizations for newly emerging or re-emerging pathogens has increased, the available technologies for production and delivery of vaccines have also increased in quality and quantity. Improved vaccine delivery methods and formulations may also contribute to vaccine safety.

With respect to emerging viral diseases of companion animals, the need for appropriate vaccines is obvious. Virus pathogens often are subject to antigenic variation [1]. Classic attenuated or inactivated vaccines may not provide sufficient antigenic diversity or developmental flexibility to meet rapidly evolving infectious threats. Also, because most viral infections are highly contagious and generally not treatable, vaccines are likely to be the most important

A contribution of the University of Nebraska Agricultural Research Division, Lincoln, NE 68583, USA.

*Corresponding author. E-mail address: dmcvey2@unl.edu (D.S. McVey).

and widely available control measure. Such considerations magnify the relative importance of vaccines for control of emerging zoonotic diseases, such as rabies.

Evidence-based data and duration of immunity suggest that the frequency of immunization can be reduced. There has also been an effort to reduce the antigenic mass of vaccines based on a definition of core sets of vaccine antigens (as determined by a relative probability of disease exposure) [1,3]. Therefore, effective clinical use of newly developed vaccines requires similar knowledge of the effective duration of immunity and a definition of the populations at risk for disease exposure. These points are addressed in this review.

RABIES VIRUS

General Comments

Rabies is a consistently progressive and fatal viral encephalitis. Closely related, neurotropic RNA viruses (family Rhabdoviridae, genus *Lyssavirus*) cause this disease [4]. Virus transmission occurs principally through animal bites. Once sufficient virus is transferred through a bite wound, the virus migrates toward central nervous tissue, followed by replication and spread to salivary glands or other peripheral sites. Because the initial centripetal transfer usually takes several days to weeks, there is opportunity for postexposure prophylaxis with vaccine or immune globulin. Rabid dogs have historically been the principal threat to human beings [5]. Successful immunization programs for dogs (and other domestic species) have nearly eliminated human rabies in North America. As new strains of rabies emerge or as other LVs emerge, however, it is critical to maintain discovery and development research to ensure sufficient immunogenicity of people and animals.

Costs of immune globulin and vaccines (particularly in underdeveloped regions of the world) prevent their use for prevention of rabies or for postexposure treatment [6]. Therefore, continued development to address these problems is warranted. Available rabies vaccines are generally efficacious against common and regional RV strains [3,7–9]. It is also clear that endemic and sporadic RV infections in wildlife are subject to long-distance translocation events, however [10,11]. Some wildlife reservoirs of LV, such as bats, may serve as sources of new RV exposure [12].

Emerging Rabies and Lyssavirus Diseases

Single-point mutations in the RV major glycoprotein (RGP) gene have resulted in increased pathogenicity because of increased viral spread within the central nervous system [13,14]. These mutations could potentially facilitate escape of host immune responses by decreasing time required for centripetal and centrifugal spread. Although these mutations were forced laboratory artifacts, it is clear that mutant strains may translocate and prove to be emerging threats. One example of newly emerging LV disease is the Australian bat Lyssavirus (ABLV) [15]. This virus is genetically and serologically distinct from RV. Conventional rabies vaccines are cross-protective in mice, however, and the standard rabies postexposure prophylaxis methods are used to treat people exposed to ABLV. Similar cross-protection has been observed in challenge of immunity experiments with other LV strains [16].

The Arctic fox strain of RV has been endemic in Ontario, Canada for several decades, and there are four dominant genetic variants. There have been incursions of a fifth variant from more northerly regions of Canada, however [17]. Nevertheless, oral vaccination over a 10-year period delivered in baits with the Evelyn-Rokitnicki-Abelseth RV has successfully controlled fox rabies in the region (96 cases in 1973–1989 and 5 cases in 1999–2006) [18]. These examples do illustrate the potential for rapid spread of new virulent mutant strains of RV and the polyvalent nature of rabies vaccines providing immunity against multiple variants of Arctic fox RV.

Although the vaccines that are currently in use demonstrate potent cross-strain immunogenicity, it cannot be assumed that this is always going to be the case. Neutralization escape mutants have been generated in vitro that are not neutralized by rabies-specific monoclonal antibodies [14]. Therefore, it is important to evaluate cross-strain protection continually and develop new antigens for vaccine use. It would also be desirable to improve the safety of rabies vaccines [19,20]. As previously mentioned, the desirability to maintain strain coverage, to improve safety by reducing risks associated with receiving rabies vaccines, and to eliminate technical barriers to availability associated with production and distribution costs justifies continued rabies vaccine development.

Rabies Vaccine Research

Rabies vaccines for companion animals have traditionally been produced in cell culture and subsequently inactivated and formulated with standard materials and processes. Use of these vaccines has had a tremendous impact on reducing rabies in dogs and cats, and therefore in human beings [4]. Even so, there have been attempts to improve these vaccines. One approach has generated recombinant RV with duplicate glycoprotein genes [21]. Serial passage followed by ultraviolet inactivation resulted in an increase in the apparent immunogenicity of this antigen. Successful development of this technology could allow increased relative potency of vaccines without increasing bulk antigen content, potentially reducing some adverse reactions.

New Approaches to Rabies Immunization

As mentioned, the rabies vaccines that are currently available are efficacious and effective for prevention of rabies in domestic animals [4]. There are no significant or broad gaps in rabies vaccine strain coverage, and immunity most likely extends to other LVs. In addition, oral vaccines, such as the vaccinia-vectored RGP recombinant vaccine, extend coverage to multiple wildlife species [12]. No one formulation provides immunity to all species, however. One recent study demonstrated the safety, immunogenicity, and efficacy (as noninferiority) of recombinant rabies vaccines in dogs [8]. In other studies the RGP expressed in canine adenovirus generated protective immunity when administered intramuscularly or intranasally in mice [22]. A similar construct of an adenovirus of chimpanzees (expressing the glycoprotein of Evelyn-Rokitnicki-Abelseth RV) induced a sustained immune response to RV and solid protection in an aerosol challenge model [23]. This experimental efficacy was achieved with one oral dose and is clinically noteworthy, because inhalation of RV leads to rapid neuronal spread of the virus from olfactory tissues [21].

Cats have become a significant source of human rabies, particularly in China and other parts of Southeast Asia. A canine adenovirus rabies vaccine (CAV2-E3Δ-RGP) was used to immunize cats by intramuscular, oral, and intranasal inoculation [24]. All routes of administration generated strong immune responses that were sustained for at least 12 months. All immunized cats survived RV challenge, and the RV challenge stimulated an anamnestic response. It is clear that the adenovirus-vectored RGP vaccines may be immunogenic and efficacious in multiple animal species, likely with coverage against multiple strains of RV and LV. In addition, these adenovirus-vectored vaccines were efficacious by the oral route. This would be advantageous for immunization of wildlife or mass populations in the face of major outbreaks.

Development of DNA vaccines for RV has progressed also. The RGP gene in a plasmid was used to immunize dogs (and mice) by the intramuscular or intranasal route [25]. Mice and dogs received a second dose of vaccine (80 and 180 days, respectively, after the initial dose). The immune response in mice was protective against challenge. These experimental vaccines were immunogenic in mice and dogs (generating neutralizing antibody). In another study, bicistronic DNA from RV and canine parvovirus (CPV) was evaluated [26]. The vaccine was immunogenic in dogs and mice and protective in mice on RV challenge. Research with RV recombinant and DNA vaccine technologies should continue, with emphasis on ease of administration to large at-risk populations (including wildlife) and safe broad virus strain and species coverage.

In addition to the research and development on RV vaccines, substantial work on passive immunization materials and procedures is being done. Panels of human monoclonal antibodies that neutralize a broad set of RV isolates have been produced and characterized [27,28]. The efficacy of these monoclonal antibodies has been evaluated [29]. The use of the human monoclonal antibodies CR57 and CR409 was protective in hamsters when administered 24 hours after RV exposure, and this efficacy was comparable with equine-origin or human-origin RV immune globulin. Further, this monoclonal antibody cocktail did not alter the immunologic response to rabies vaccine (typically administered as postexposure prophylaxis). A monoclonal Fab library has been constructed that could potentially lead to broad strain coverage [30]. Production of RV-neutralizing and protective antibody in hens' eggs has been achieved, and this could also be a useful approach to provide a more affordable alternative to human or equine immunoglobulin [31]. The use of immunoglobulins could be considered for any exposed animal or for broad population exposure by means of an aerosol (as with terrorism).

PARVOVIRUS

General Comments

Parvoviruses are small nonenveloped DNA viruses that cause life-threatening infections of cats and dogs. Vaccination has provided important, although imperfect, control of these infections [2]. CPV type 2 (CPV-2) has emerged in dogs since 1978. Feline parvovirus (FPV) is responsible for panleukopenia in cats, a devastating gastroenteritis of kittens. Parvovirus vaccines for companion mammals are typically administered as components of larger polyvalent formulations. Most of these vaccines are attenuated or inactivated vaccines. Vaccination of kittens and puppies has been considered safe and effective [3,32,33]. Some concerns of safety exist, but true reversion to virulence is rare [34], and the presence of adventitious agents is also rare [35].

Two antigenically distinct strains distributed throughout the world exist: CPV-2a and CPV-2b [36]. Diagnostic tools have been developed based on the TaqMAN polymerase chain reaction to distinguish between type 2 field strains and vaccine strains [37]. Until recently, vaccine strains were type 2a, but new vaccine strains of type 2b have been developed and are available for clinical use. Type 2c strains have emerged in Europe, Vietnam, and the United States [36,38]. DNA detection and antibody detection tools are available for recognition of type 2c variants [37]. It is not clear if the emergence of type 2c variants is, at least in part, attributable to antigenic variation or immune escape [36].

New type 2b CPV vaccines are now available commercially in Europe [37]. In addition, attenuated type 2b virus has been evaluated as a potential intranasal vaccine. These experimental vaccines were immunogenic in puppies even in the face of substantial maternal antibody [39]. A polycistronic DNA vaccine for RV and CPV was immunogenic [26]. CPV-2a and CPV-2b have been isolated from cats, and the CPV-2b strain FP84 is virulent in cats. Attenuated FPV vaccines do afford protection in cats against CPV, and inactivated FPV vaccine may provide at least limited protection [40].

Clearly, new and virulent variants of CPV and FPV are generated that may have potential to escape immune responses. Therefore, continued vaccine research and development are necessary. Emphasis for development of future PV vaccines should be directed toward maximizing strain polyvalency in several animal species with technologies that also enhance safety and minimize barriers to manufacturing, distribution, and delivery.

FELINE CALICIVIRUS

General Comments

FCV is a common pathogen of cats and is primarily associated with respiratory tract disease. A member of the *Vesivirus* genus of the Caliciviridae, the small nonenveloped virus has a single-stranded linear RNA genome of positive polarity. This highly contagious virus is easily spread by direct and indirect transmission. Fomites, in particular, are an important means of spread because of environmental stability [41]. The virus replicates in the oral and respiratory tissues, and disease typically manifests as serous conjunctivitis, nasal discharge, mild upper respiratory signs, and fever [41]. A hallmark of FCV infection is ulceration of the tongue, hard palate, and nose. Most infections are mild and self-limiting. After clinical recovery, however, infection with shedding in oropharyngeal secretions may persist for periods of week to months, even in vaccinated cats [42,43].

Recently, several outbreaks of a highly virulent form of FCV have been reported [44–48]. Disease manifestations in these outbreaks have included high fever; depression; anorexia; edema, particularly of the head and limbs; and ulcerative dermatitis of the face, pinnae, and feet. Systemic involvement with multiorgan dysfunction (lungs, pancreas, and liver) may occur. In most of these occurrences, the index case originated from a shelter or rescue facility. Vaccinated and unvaccinated cats have been affected, with significant mortality rates [44–49]. An immune-mediated pathogenesis may be at least partially responsible for the lesions in virulent systemic disease (VSD) [50]. Experimental evidence indicates that the virus is capable of causing disease without cofactors [44]. The specific viral factor(s) responsible for this virulent phenotype have not been identified, however. Viral molecular markers have not been found. The mutation or mutations responsible seem to evolve independently in each outbreak, and isolates from VSD episodes characterized thus far are distinct from one another [44–47,50].

The FCV genome encodes a single major structural protein that forms the capsid [48]. This protein has been divided into six regions based on sequence analysis [49,51–53]. Among these regions, designated A through F, C and E have significant variability (20%–40%); in particular, hypervariable regions of the E region have been identified, with genetic distances as high as 68% between unrelated isolates [18,19]. These regions have been used for molecular epidemiology [52,54]. In addition, they contain immunodominant neutralizing epitopes [55–57]. As a result, there is significant antigenic variability among FCV isolates. This variability may have evolved as a result of immune selection [52,54,58,59]. Isolates from FCV infections of vaccinated cats vary significantly, which may be responsible for vaccine failures [52,54].

Persistent infections after recovery from acute disease are not uncommon. Infected cats may continue to shed the virus throughout their lifetime, but most shed for periods of weeks to a few months [41]. In addition, reinfection from within infected populations, even with closely related variants, occurs regularly [60]. Strains circulating in endemically injected colonies may vary as much as 19% in the variable regions of the capsid protein [53]. Endemically infected colonies may provide an environment for increasing FCV genetic (and thus antigenic) diversity and may lead to the emergence of new strains with varying virulence [42,61]. In an isolated population of cats, emergence of antigenically distinct strains has been documented [62]. The possibility exists that new disease phenotypes could also emerge in infected populations.

Feline Calicivirus Immunity

Strains of FCV, including the virulent systemic strains, differ in their ability to be neutralized by antibody produced against heterologous strains [44,58,62].

This variability creates a challenge for development of efficacious vaccines. Despite the use of vaccines using strains of FCV that have relatively broad cross-reactivity (eg, F9 strain, 255 strain) infection and disease may still occur in vaccinated cats. The outbreak of virulent systemic FCV in vaccinated cats is a recent example [41].

Manufacturers are investigating the utility of including additional strains in vaccines to increase the spectrum of protection. At least one manufacturer (Ft. Dodge Laboratories, Fort Dodge, Iowa) has licensed an FCV vaccine with extended strain coverage. Ideally, these strains should increase the antigenic heterogeneity of the vaccine. Synergy among heterologous strains to stimulate a more cross-protective response has been shown [63]. Because of the strain variability, however, it is difficult to achieve a vaccine that provides protection to all strains in circulation. A study by Hohdatsu and colleagues [64] found that although immunization with more than one strain increased the cross-neutralizing activity of the antibody response, 22% to 44% of the isolates tested still were not neutralized. Thus, there is significant variation in neutralizing antigenicity between vaccinal and circulating wild strains. In addition, antigenic clustering does not correlate with disease manifestation [65]. Thus, inclusion of two or more strains isolated from different disease manifestations does not necessarily ensure broad protection against the varied pathogenic phenotypes.

Current FCV vaccines do not protect against infection but do protect against developing disease [41]. In addition, they may not eliminate the carrier state or prevent episodes of reinfection [42,61]. Combining FCV strains or isolates in single vaccines may prove to be useful for increasing the efficacy of vaccines. Strains to be used for vaccine must be carefully selected, however, based on analysis of their nucleotide and antigenic properties (including the range of important epitopes that are required). Synergy with the combination of isolates must be demonstrated to substantiate claims of broad antigenic protection [62,63]. Alternatively, as key antigenic epitopes are characterized, recombinant technology may allow development of vaccines with a broad spectrum of protection. For example, recombinant vector vaccines expressing multiple or conserved epitopes may be designed. A recombinant vector vaccine developed by McCabe and Spibey [66] incorporated capsid genes of two distinct strains, increasing the antigenic spectrum. DNA vaccines have also been used experimentally to induce protection against disease [67]. In addition, subunit vaccines containing capsids of the virus have had some success [68]. At least for the foreseeable future, however, FCV is likely to continue to be an important pathogen in cats, despite advances in vaccine development.

CANINE DISTEMPER

General Comments

Canine distemper virus (CDV) is a significant pathogen of dogs that has affected Canidae for thousands of years [69]. The virus, a member of the genus *Morbillivirus* in the family Paramyxoviridae, infects domestic dogs and a wide variety of carnivores. The virus is highly contagious, is shed in all secretions, and is spread by direct contact and by indirect transmission by means of aerosol. Infection may lead to a multisystemic disease. The genome is encased in a helical capsid, which is surrounded by a lipid envelope. This last characteristic makes the virus relatively labile in the environment, and it remains viable for only a few hours at room temperature; however, at freezing temperature, it may persist for several weeks [69]. Embedded in the envelope are glycoproteins F (fusion) and H (hemagglutinin [HA]), which are important antigens of the virus. They contain important immunodominant epitopes and are major antigen targets for the host immune response [65,70]. In addition, they affect the tissue tropism of the virus [71].

As with other RNA viruses, strains of CDV vary genetically. The gene encoding the H protein has the greatest genetic diversity and allows discrimination of the various CDV lineages [72–74]. This gene segregates six major genetic CDV lineages: America-1 and -2, Asia-1 and -2, European, and Arctic [75]. Many commercial vaccines include strains from the America-1 lineage (eg, Snyder Hill, Onderstepoort, Lederle), although these genotypes do not seem to be circulating in the field currently [75]. Novel CDV strains have been identified in recent years throughout the world. Outbreaks with some strains may have been translocated from distant geographic locales. For example, the Arctic lineage occurs in Italy, and isolates from dogs in Hungary resemble those from North America [74,76]. This may occur as a consequence of extensive and often uncontrolled movement and trade of dogs and exchange of CDV strains with wildlife, such as raccoons.

Distinct isolates have also been detected in North America. In 2004, phylogenetic analysis of virus from four clinical cases identified three strains genetically distant from strains previously identified in North America [77]. The dogs in three of these four cases had recently been vaccinated. Genetic characterization of the viruses from these cases found that they were novel for the continental United States. Circulation in wildlife populations may lead to viruses varying in antigenicity and virulence. CDV in dogs may result from contact with wildlife. An outbreak of canine distemper in Alaska led to the death of several hundred dogs [78]. The virus was isolated and characterized and was most closely related to a Phocine distemper virus from an outbreak among Baikul seals in Siberia. In Africa, infection leading to disease and death among lions is believed to have originated from domestic dogs from villages neighboring the wildlife preserves [79,80]. Infection in stone martens and foxes in Germany has been reported [81], and in the United States, based on seroprevalence, raccoons are often infected in periurban regions. Raccoons may have transmitted the virus to captive felids in an urban zoo and may have been the source of virus in a Chicago area outbreak among domestic dogs [82,83].

Vaccination to Prevent Canine Distemper Virus Disease

The advent of vaccination for CDV in the 1950s led to a decrease in the incidence of distemper in dogs [84]. Most vaccines are attenuated-live vaccines.

Adverse reactions from vaccination have been reported, including inclusion body encephalitis [85]. Reversion to virulence is a concern but is not a frequent cause of distemper. This concern is avoided with the advent of recombinant vaccines for CDV that are now available. These vaccines incorporate the genes for the envelope glycoproteins in a canarypox vector [86,87], and immunity to CDV is induced without the risk for intact live CDV. The antibody response and protection afforded by this vaccine are similar to those of modified-live virus (MLV) [86,87]. DNA vaccines also have been developed and may not be affected by maternal immunity [88]. A DNA plasmid expressing the nucleocapsid protein and the surface proteins H and F induced a significant priming effect in 14-day-old pups despite high titers of maternal antibodies. Furthermore, a DNA plasmid incorporating the H and F protein genes induced solid protection to homologous challenge [89]. These new vaccine strategies may lead to improved CDV vaccines.

The major concern with current vaccines is efficacy. The disease still occurs throughout the world, and outbreaks in vaccinated dogs have been reported. Genetic diversity has been associated with vaccine failures. Unique strains have been associated with infections of vaccinated dogs in Mexico, and, phylogenetically, these isolates were most closely related to isolates from Germany [70]. In Japan, infection of vaccinated dogs with isolates from the Asia-1 group distantly related to vaccine strains have been documented [90]. Also, distantly related to the vaccine virus group was a CDV strain from the Asia-2 group isolated from a diseased dog that had been vaccinated against CDV [91].

As new strains of CDV continue to emerge, surveillance and characterization of isolates from field cases are necessary. Antigenic, pathogenic, and genotypic descriptions of new isolates should provide important information about this important pathogen required to maintain safe and efficacious vaccines.

INFLUENZA
General Comments
In January 2004, an outbreak of respiratory disease occurred in racing greyhounds in Florida [92]. Although some animals exhibited mild disease, others developed severe pneumonia, with a case fatality rate of 36%. Virus isolations on postmortem samples resulted in identification of an influenza virus. The virus was similar to equine influenza virus A (H3N8). Archived sera were subsequently tested for antibodies and revealed evidence of infection in dogs as far back as 2000. Evidence of infection has also been observed in several geographic regions of the United States among shelter and pet dogs in addition to racing greyhounds.

Influenza virus is a member of the Orthomyxoviridae, a single-stranded RNA virus whose genome is segmented. Subtypes are distinguished by antigenicity of the envelope glycoproteins HA and neuraminidase (NA). The virus is relatively labile in the environment but is highly contagious and easily spread by aerosol. Influenza viruses affect several terrestrial and marine mammals in addition to birds. The virus targets epithelia of the respiratory tract, and in birds, it targets the enteric tract [93,94].

The genomic properties of influenza virus allow not only for intramolecular mutations as is commonly seen with RNA viruses but for reassortment of gene segments between viruses infecting the same cell. When these mutations involve the surface glycoproteins, antigenic drift and shift, respectively, occur. This ability for subtle and major changes in antigenicity makes immunization against influenza difficult.

Although the first characterization of this virus in dogs was from an outbreak with significant mortality, it seems that most uncomplicated infections are relatively mild [95,96]. After an incubation of 2 to 5 days, most dogs have symptoms similar to kennel cough, with moist cough, fever, and nasal discharge. Because most dogs are immunologically naive to influenza, adults and puppies may be susceptible to infection [95]. Secondary bacterial infections can lead to severe pneumonia in infected animals regardless of age [96], however. Morbidity approaches 100% in some outbreaks [96]. A peracute form with hemorrhage in the respiratory tract may occur in a few infections [95]. The transmission of equine influenza to dogs was an uncommon occurrence of interspecies spread of an intact virus without reassortment. From viral analyses of subsequent occurrences, it seems that this was a single interspecies transfer of virus attributable to point mutations rather than to reassortment of gene segments [95].

Mucosal and systemic immunity are important in protection against influenza [97]. Protection against infection with influenza is mediated primarily by antibodies to the surface antigens and includes mucosal and serum immunoglobulin [97]. Cell-mediated immunity (CMI) is also important and seems to function mainly in recovery and clearance of the virus [98]. The antigen targets that induce the CMI are often more conserved than those of humoral immunity [99].

Currently, no vaccines are available for canine influenza, and the equine influenza vaccines should not be used in dogs. Several vaccines are in development, however, and are expected to become available in the near future. Killed, subunit, or live vaccines may be used. In addition, recombinant live vector vaccines may become available, and intranasal and parenteral administration may be used, depending on the vaccine types.

The killed whole-virus vaccines and subunit vaccines containing viral proteins primarily induce humoral immunity because there is no vaccinal virus replication. For influenza virus, protective neutralizing antibodies target the surface glycoproteins [97]. Because of the potential for antigenic variation in these proteins, updating of human vaccines occurs annually. It is not known if the canine influenza virus has a similar propensity for change.

Mucosal influenza vaccines are available for human beings, horses, and birds, and they may be used for canine influenza. These live-attenuated vaccines induce a secretory and systemic response. In addition, this immune response is mediated not only by the humoral arm but by the cell-mediated arm of the immune system. The result may more closely mimic natural infection, which is known to induce a long-lived immunity [99]. Recombinant live canarypox vector vaccine expressing the HA antigen of influenza is available for horses. This vaccine also induces both arms of the immune response, although avoiding the risk for live influenza virus [99].

Before a new vaccine for canine influenza can be recommended, it is necessary to investigate the epidemiology of this virus, including the pathogenicity, transmissibility, and incidence and prevalence of infections. It is likely that vaccination of dogs at high risk, such as in shelter situations or boarding kennels, would be recommended. The vaccine choice would depend on independent efficacy studies.

SUMMARY

It is likely that new viral disease may continue to emerge in companion animals (eg, that caused by influenza or LV encephalitis). It is more likely that genetic or antigenic virus variants or geographically translocated viruses may emerge or re-emerge in companion animals (eg, RV, CDV, CPV, FCV), however. This latter possibility represents the greater risk. Because this represents an ongoing threat, research and development should continue to maximize broad efficacy and effectiveness in addition to safety. To achieve these goals, the research and development effort should evaluate newer available technologies that may also reduce any barriers to use and availability.

References

  [1] Meeusen ENT, Walker J, Peters A, et al. Current status of veterinary vaccines. Clin Microbiol Rev 2007;20(3):489–510.
  [2] Schultz RD. Duration of immunity for canine and feline vaccines: a review. Vet Microbiol 2006;117(1):75–9.
  [3] Lakshmanan N, Gore TC, Duncan KL, et al. Three-year rabies duration of immunity in dogs following vaccination with a core combination vaccine against canine distemper virus, canine adenovirus type-1, canine parvovirus, and rabies virus. Vet Ther 2006;7(3):223–31.
  [4] Rupprecht CE, Hanlon CA, Hemachudha T. Rabies re-examined. Lancet Infect Dis 2002;2(6):327–43.
  [5] Zinsstag J, Schelling E, Roth F, et al. Human benefits of animal interventions for zoonosis control. Emerg Infect Dis 2007;13(4):527–31.
  [6] Wilde H, Khawplod P, Khamoltham T, et al. Rabies control in South and Southeast Asia. Vaccine 2005;23(17–18):2284–9.
  [7] Sidwa TJ, Wilson PJ, Moore GM, et al. Evaluation of oral rabies vaccination programs for control of rabies epizootics in coyotes and gray foxes: 1995–2003. J Am Vet Med Assoc 2005;227(5):785–92.
  [8] Rupprecht CE, Hanlon CA, Blanton J, et al. Oral vaccination of dogs with recombinant rabies virus vaccines. Virus Res 2005;111(1):101–5.
  [9] Rupprecht CE, Hanlon CA, Slate D. Oral vaccination of wildlife against rabies: opportunities and challenges in prevention and control. Dev Biol 2004;119:173–84.
  [10] Russell CA, Smith DL, Childs JE, et al. Predictive spatial dynamics and strategic planning for raccoon rabies emergence in Ohio. PLoS Biol 2005;3(3):e88.
  [11] Russell CA, Real LA, Smith DL. Spatial control of rabies on heterogeneous landscapes. PLoS ONE 2006;1:e27.
  [12] Hanlon CA, Kuzmin IV, Blanton JD, et al. Efficacy of rabies biologics against new Lyssaviruses from Eurasia. Virus Res 2005;111(1):44–54.

[13] Faber M, Faber ML, Papaneri A, et al. A single amino acid change in rabies virus glycoprotein increases virus spread and enhances virus pathogenicity. J Virol 2005;79(22):14141–8.

[14] Marissen WE, Kramer RA, Rice A, et al. Novel rabies virus-neutralizing epitope recognized by human monoclonal antibody: fine mapping and escape mutant analysis. J Virol 2005;79(8):4672–8.

[15] Warrilow D. Australian bat Lyssavirus: a recently discovered new rhabdovirus. Curr Top Microbiol Immunol 2005;292:25–44.

[16] Müller T, Selhorst T, Burow J, et al. Cross reactive antigenicity in orally vaccinated foxes and raccoon dogs against European Bat Lyssavirus type 1 and 2. Dev Biol 2006;125:195–204.

[17] Nadin-Davis SA, Muldoon F, Wandeler AI. Persistence of genetic variants of the Arctic fox strain of rabies virus in southern Ontario. Can J Vet Res 2006;70(1):11–9.

[18] Rosatte RC, Power MJ, Donovan D, et al. Elimination of Arctic variant rabies in red foxes, metropolitan Toronto. Emerg Infect Dis 2007;13(1):25–7.

[19] Moore GE, Ward MP, Kulldorff M, et al. A space-time cluster of adverse events associated with canine rabies vaccine. Vaccine 2005;23(48–49):5557–62.

[20] Rasalingam P, Rossiter JP, Jackson AC. Recombinant rabies virus vaccine strain SAD-l16 inoculated intracerebrally in young mice produces a severe encephalitis with extensive neuronal apoptosis. Can J Vet Res 2005;69(2):100–5.

[21] Hosokawa-Muto J, Ito N, Yamada K, et al. Characterization of recombinant rabies virus carrying double glycoprotein genes. Microbiol Immunol 2006;50(3):187–96.

[22] Li J, Faber M, Papaneri A, et al. A single immunization with a recombinant canine adenovirus expressing the rabies virus G protein confers protective immunity against rabies in mice. Virology 2006;356(1–2):147–54.

[23] Zhou D, Cun A, Li Y, et al. A chimpanzee-origin adenovirus vector expressing the rabies virus glycoprotein as an oral vaccine against inhalation infection with rabies virus. Mol Ther 2006;14(5):662–72.

[24] Hu RL, Liu Y, Zhang SF, et al. Experimental immunization of cats with a recombinant rabies-canine adenovirus vaccine elicits a long-lasting neutralizing antibody response against rabies. Vaccine 2007;25(29):5301–7.

[25] Tesoro Cruz E, Hernández González R, Alonso Morales R, et al. Rabies DNA vaccination by the intranasal route in dogs. Dev Biol 2006;125:221–31.

[26] Patial S, Chaturvedi VK, Rai A, et al. Virus neutralizing antibody response in mice and dogs with a bicistronic DNA vaccine encoding rabies virus glycoprotein and canine parvovirus VP2. Vaccine 2007;25(20):4020–8.

[27] Sloan SE, Hanlon C, Weldon W, et al. Identification and characterization of a human monoclonal antibody that potently neutralizes a broad panel of rabies virus isolates. Vaccine 2007;25(15):2800–10.

[28] de Kruif J, Bakker AB, Marissen WE, et al. A human monoclonal antibody cocktail as a novel component of rabies postexposure prophylaxis. Annu Rev Med 2007;58:359–68.

[29] Goudsmit J, Marissen WE, Weldon WC, et al. Comparison of an anti-rabies human monoclonal antibody combination with human polyclonal anti-rabies immune globulin. J Infect Dis 2006;193(6):796–801.

[30] Ando T, Yamashiro T, Takita-Sonoda Y, et al. Construction of human Fab library and isolation of monoclonal Fabs with rabies virus-neutralizing ability. Microbiol Immunol 2005;49(4):311–22.

[31] Motoi Y, Sato K, Hatta H, et al. Production of rabies neutralizing antibody in hens' eggs using a part of the G protein expressed in Escherichia coli. Vaccine 2005;23(23):3026–32.

[32] Jacobs AA, Bergman JG, Theelen RP, et al. Compatibility of a bivalent modified-live vaccine against Bordetella bronchiseptica and CPiV, and a trivalent modified-live vaccine against CPV, CDV and CAV-2. Vet Rec 2007;160(2):41–5.

[33] Gore TC, Lakshmanan N, Duncan KL, et al. Three-year duration of immunity in dogs following vaccination against canine adenovirus type-1, canine parvovirus, and canine distemper virus. Vet Ther 2005;6(1):5–14.

[34] Decaro N, Desario C, Elia G, et al. Occurrence of severe gastroenteritis in pups after canine parvovirus vaccine administration: a clinical and laboratory diagnostic dilemma. Vaccine 2007;25(7):1161–6.
[35] Nims RW. Detection of adventitious viruses in biologicals—a rare occurrence. Dev Biol 2006;123:153–64 [discussion: 183–97].
[36] Decaro N, Desario C, Addie DD, et al. Molecular epidemiology of canine parvovirus, Europe. Emerg Infect Dis 2007;13(8):1222–4.
[37] Decaro N, Martella V, Elia G, et al. Diagnostic tools based on minor groove binder probe technology for rapid identification of vaccinal and field strains of canine parvovirus type 2b. J Virol Methods 2006;138(1–2):10–6.
[38] Kapil S, Cooper E, Lamm C, et al. Canine parvovirus types 2c and 2b circulating in North American dogs in 2006 and 2007. J Clin Microbiol 2007;45(12):4044–7.
[39] Martella V, Cavalli A, Decaro N, et al. Immunogenicity of an intranasally administered modified live canine parvovirus type 2b vaccine in pups with maternally derived antibodies. Clin Diagn Lab Immunol 2005;12(10):1243–5.
[40] Gamoh K, Senda M, Inoue Y, et al. Efficacy of an inactivated feline panleucopenia virus vaccine against a canine parvovirus isolated from a domestic cat. Vet Rec 2005;157(10):285–7.
[41] Radford AD, Coyne KP, Dawson S, et al. Feline calicivirus. Vet Res 2007;38(2):319–35.
[42] Pedersen NC, Hawkins KF. Mechanisms for persistence of acute and chronic feline calicivirus infections in the face of vaccination. Vet Microbiol 1995;47(1–2):141–56.
[43] Wardley RC. Feline calicivirus carrier state: a study of the host/virus relationship. Arch Virol 1976;52:243–9.
[44] Pedersen NC, Elliot JB, Glasgow A, et al. An isolated epizootic of hemorrhagic-like fever in cats caused by a novel and highly virulent strain of feline calicivirus. Vet Microbiol 2000;73(4):281–300.
[45] Abd-Eldaim M, Potgieter L, Kennedy M. Genetic analysis of feline caliciviruses associated with a hemorrhagic-like disease. J Vet Diagn Invest 2005;17(5):420–9.
[46] Hurley KF, Pesavento PA, Pedersen NC, et al. An outbreak of virulent systemic feline calicivirus disease. J Am Vet Med Assoc 2004;224(2):241–9.
[47] Rong S, Slade D, Floyd Hawkins K, et al. Characterization of a highly virulent feline calicivirus and attenuation of this virus. Virus Res 2006;122(1–2):95–108.
[48] Thiel HJ, Konig M. Caliciviruses: an overview. Vet Microbiol 1999;69(1–2):55–62.
[49] Glenn M, Radford AD, Turner PC, et al. Nucleotide sequence of UK and Australian isolates of feline calicivirus (FCV) and phylogenetic analysis of FCVs. Vet Microbiol 1999;67(3):175–93.
[50] Foley J, Hurley K, Pesavento PA, et al. Virulent systemic feline calicivirus infection: local cytokine modulation and contribution of viral mutants. J Feline Med Surg 2006;8(1):55–61.
[51] Seal BS, Ridpath JF, Mengeling WL. Analysis of feline calicivirus capsid protein genes—identification of variable antigenic determinant regions of the protein. J Gen Virol 1993;74:2519–24.
[52] Radford AD, Bennett M, McArdle F, et al. The use of sequence analysis of a feline calicivirus (FCV) hypervariable region in the epidemiological investigation of FCV related disease and vaccine failures. Vaccine 1997;15(12–13):1451–8.
[53] Radford AD, Bennett M, McArdle F, et al. High genetic diversity of the immunodominant region of the feline calicivirus capsid gene in endemically infected cat colonies. Virus Genes 2003;27(2):145–55.
[54] Radford AD, Dawson S, Wharmby C, et al. Comparison of serological and sequence-based methods for typing feline calicivirus isolates from vaccine failures. Vet Rec 2000;146(5):117–23.
[55] Geissler K, Schneider K, Truyen U. Mapping neutralizing and non-neutralizing epitopes on the capsid protein of feline calicivirus. J Vet Med B Infect Dis Vet Public Health 2002;49(1):55–60.

[56] Tohya Y, Yokoyama N, Maes K, et al. Mapping of antigenic sites involved in neutralization on the capsid protein of feline calicivirus. J Gen Virol 1997;78:303–5.

[57] Radfor AD, Willoughby K, Dawson S, et al. The capsid gene of feline calicivirus contains linear B-cell epitopes in both variable and conserved regions. J Virol 1999;73(10):8496–502.

[58] Kreutz LC, Johnson RP, Seal BS. Phenotypic and genotypic variation of feline calicivirus during persistent infection of cats. Vet Microbiol 1998;59(2–3):229–36.

[59] Nilsson M, Hedlund KO, Thorhagen M, et al. Evolution of human calicivirus RNA in vivo: accumulation of mutations in the protruding P2 domain of the capsid leads to structural changes and possibly a new phenotype. J Virol 2003;77(24):13117–24.

[60] Coyne KP, Gaskell RM, Dawson S, et al. Evolutionary mechanisms of persistence and diversification of a calicivirus within endemically infected natural host populations. J Virol 2007;81(4):1961–71.

[61] Coyne KP, Reed FC, Porter CJ, et al. Recombination of feline calicivirus within an endemically infected cat colony. J Gen Virol 2006;87:921–6.

[62] Johnson RP. Antigenic change in feline calicivirus during persistent infection. Can J Vet Res 1992;56(4):326–30.

[63] Poulet H, Brunet S, Leroy V, et al. Immunisation with a combination of two complementary feline calicivirus strains induces a broad cross-protection against heterologous challenges. Vet Microbiol 2005;106(1–2):17–31.

[64] Hohdatsu T, Sato K, Tajima T, et al. Neutralizing feature of commercially available feline calicivirus (FCV) vaccine immune sera against FCV field isolates. J Vet Med Sci 1999;61(3):299–301.

[65] Poulet H, Togashi K, Wakasa C, et al. Comparison between acute oral/respiratory and chronic stomatitis/gingivitis isolates of feline calicivirus: pathogenicity, antigenic profile and cross-neutralisation studies. Archives of Virology 2000;145(2):243–61.

[66] McCabe VJ, Spibey NN. Potential for broad-spectrum protection against feline calicivirus using an attenuated myxoma virus expressing a chimeric FCV capsid protein. Vaccine 2005;23(46–47):5380–8.

[67] Sommerville LM, Radford AD, Glenn M, et al. DNA vaccination against feline calicivirus infection using a plasmid encoding the mature capsid protein. Vaccine 2002;20(13–14):1787–96.

[68] Di Martino B, Marsilio F, Roy P. Assembly of feline calicivirus-like particle and its immunogenicity. Vet Microbiol 2007;120(1–2):173–8.

[69] Deem SL, Spelman LH, Yates RA, et al. Canine distemper in terrestrial carnivores: a review. J Zoo Wildl Med 2000;31(4):441–51.

[70] Simon-Martinez J, Ulloa-Arvizu R, Soriano VE, et al. Identification of a genetic variation of canine distemper virus from clinical cases in two vaccinated dogs in Mexico. Vet J 2008;175(3):423–6.

[71] von Messling V, Fielding A, Cattaneo R. Of dogs and men: canine distemper virus as model system for measles virus. Gene Therapy 2001;8:S13.

[72] Haas L, Lierman HL, Harder TC, et al. Analysis of the haemagglutinin gene of current wild-type canine distemper virus isolates from Germany. Virus Res 1997;48(1997):165–71.

[73] Iwatsuki K, Miyashita N, Yoshid E, et al. Molecular and phylogenetic analyses of the haemagglutinin (H) proteins of field isolates of canine distemper virus from naturally infected dogs. J Gen Virol 1997;78:373–80.

[74] Martella V, Cirone F, Elia G, et al. Heterogeneity within the hemagglutinin genes of canine distemper virus (CDV) strains detected in Italy. Vet Microbiol 2006;116(4):301–9.

[75] Martella V, Elia G, Lucente MS, et al. Genotyping canine distemper virus (CDV) by a heminested multiplex PCR provides a rapid approach for investigation of CDV outbreaks. Vet Microbiol 2007;122(1–2):32–42.

[76] Demeter Z, Lakatos B, Palade EA, et al. Genetic diversity of Hungarian canine distemper virus strains. Vet Microbiol 2007;122(3–4):258–69.

[77] Pardo IDR, Johnson GC, Kleiboeker SB. Phylogenetic characterization of canine distemper viruses detected in naturally infected dogs in North America. J Clin Microbiol 2005;43(10): 5009–17.

[78] Maes RK, Wise AG, Fitzgerald SD, et al. A canine distemper outbreak in Alaska: diagnosis and strain characterization using sequence analysis. J Vet Diagn Invest 2003;15(3): 213–20.

[79] Evermann JF, Leathers CW, Gorham JR. Pathogenesis of two strains of lion (Panthera leo) Morbillivirus in ferrets (Mustela putorius furo). Vet Pathol 2001;38(3):311–6.

[80] Evermann JF, McKeirnan AJ, Gorham JR. Interspecies virus transmission. Compendium on Continuing Education for the Practicing Veterinarian 2002;24(5):390–7.

[81] Frolich K, Streich WJ, Fickel J, et al. Epizootiological investigations of canine distemper virus in free-ranging carnivores from Germany. Vet Microbiol 2000;74(4):283–92.

[82] Junge RE, et al. A serologic assessment of exposure to viral pathogens and Leptospira in an urban raccoon (Procyon lotor) population inhabiting a large zoological park. J Zoo Wildl Med 2007;38(1):18–26.

[83] Kuehn BM. Multidisciplinary task force tackles Chicago distemper outbreak. J Am Vet Med Assoc 2004;1315–7.

[84] Chappuis G. Control of canine-distemper. Vet Microbiol 1995;44(2–4):351–8.

[85] Hirayama N, et al. Protective effects of monoclonal-antibodies against lethal canine-distemper virus-infection in mice. J Gen Virol 1991;72:2827–30.

[86] Larson LJ, Schultz RD. Effect of vaccination with recombinant canine distemper virus vaccine immediately before exposure under shelter-like conditions. Vet Ther 2006;7(2):113–8.

[87] Larson LJ, Hageny TL, Hasse CJ, et al. Effect of recombinant canine distemper vaccine on antibody titers in previously vaccinated dogs. Vet Ther 2006;7(2):107–12.

[88] Griot C, Moser C, Cherpillod P, et al. Early DNA vaccination of puppies against canine dis-temper in the presence of maternally derived immunity. Vaccine 2004;22(5–6):650–4.

[89] Fischer L, Tronel JP, Minke J, et al. Vaccination of puppies with a lipid-formulated plasmid vaccine protects against a severe canine distemper virus challenge. Vaccine 2003;21(11–12):1099–102.

[90] Lan NT, Yamaguchi R, Inomata A, et al. Comparative analyses of canine distemper viral iso-lates from clinical cases of canine distemper in vaccinated dogs. Vet Microbiol 2006;115(1–3):32–42.

[91] Lan NT, Yamaguchi R, Furuya Y, et al. Pathogenesis and phylogenetic analyses of canine distemper virus strain 007Lm, a new isolate in dogs. Vet Microbiol 2005;110(3–4): 197–207.

[92] Crawford PC, Dubovi E, Castleman WL, et al. Transmission of equine influenza virus to dogs. Science 2005;310:482–5.

[93] Yamamoto Y, Nakamura K, Kitagawa K, et al. Severe nonpurulent encephalitis with mortal-ity and feather lesions in call ducks (Anas platyrhyncha var. domestica) inoculated intrave-nously with H5N1 highly pathogenic avian influenza virus. Avian Dis 2007;51(1):52–7.

[94] Studahl M. Influenza virus and CNS manifestations. J Clin Virol 2003;28(3):225–32.

[95] Buonavoglia C, Martella V. Canine respiratory viruses. Vet Res 2007;38(2007):355–73.

[96] Yoon KJ, Cooper VL, Schwartz KJ, et al. Influenza virus infection in racing greyhounds. Emerg Infect Dis 2005;11(12):1974–6.

[97] Cox RJ, Brokstad KA, Ogra P. Influenza virus: immunity and vaccination strategies, comparison of the immune response to inactivated and live, attenuated influenza vaccines. Scand J Immunol 2004;59:1–15.

[98] Thomas PG, Keating R, Hulse-Post DJ, et al. Cell-mediated protection in influenza infection. Emerg Infect Dis 2006;12(1):48–54.

[99] Daly JM, Newton JR, Mumford JA. Current perspectives on control of equine influenza. Vet Res 2004;35(2004):411–23.

Vet Clin Small Anim 38 (2008) 919–929

VETERINARY CLINICS
SMALL ANIMAL PRACTICE

Accidental Introduction of Viruses into Companion Animals by Commercial Vaccines

James F. Evermann, PhD

Department of Veterinary Clinical Sciences, Washington Animal Disease Diagnostic Laboratory, College of Veterinary Medicine, Washington State University, Pullman, WA 99164, USA

> Nevertheless, we can be confident that all future viruses will arise from those now existent: they will be mutants, recombinants, and reassortments [1].

Vaccination of dogs and cats has been regarded as one of the major success stories in veterinary medicine. Originally, the use of vaccines was to provide a barrier to infectious agents, such as rabies, that were known to be transmitted between dogs and human beings [2]. As public health concerns were addressed, the use of vaccines to control infectious diseases that cause high morbidity or high morality were then included in vaccination programs [3–6]. Vaccination has been proved to be the most efficient and cost-effective method of controlling the major infectious diseases in domestic animals [7,8]. Although we do not normally consider vaccination as way for an animal to become infected with a microorganism, it was originally intended for this purpose—a planned infection with a known infectious dose of nonlethal consequences. Later, vaccines with attenuated (modified) microorganisms that induced a sustained protective immune response with minimal side effects were used [7–10].

The key objective of this article is the recognition of the fact that the use of vaccines is not without risks and what clinicians can do to assist in the recognition and reporting of such adverse events. The main focus is on contamination of vaccines, the types of contaminants, and the effects on vaccinated animals.

PRINCIPLES AND TYPES OF VACCINATION

There are three types of vaccine strategies used in veterinary medicine [11]. These include (1) routine vaccination of susceptible animals to maintain "herd immunity" against endemic or established infections in an area; (2) strategic vaccination that uses emergency vaccination, ring vaccination, and barrier vaccination; and (3) suppressive or dampening-down vaccination. The primary type of vaccination used in companion animals is routine vaccination, because

E-mail address: jfe@vetmed.wsu.edu

0195-5616/08/$ – see front matter
doi:10.1016/j.cvsm.2008.02.010

disease prevention in an individual animal is the objective. Forms of strategic vaccination are used in areas that are trying to control infectious diseases in populations, such as in kennels or catteries, however [8]. A further division in vaccines has been the labeling of vaccines based on their clinical importance [4,7]. Essential, or core, vaccines are those vaccines that are recommended to be administered routinely to dogs and cats to protect them against endemic diseases that have high morbidity or mortality rates. Optional, or noncore, vaccines are those vaccines that are not recommended to be used routinely because the disease risk is considered to be lower. It should be emphasized that noncore does not mean nonessential, however, because certain animal populations are at high risk for disease, such as canine coronavirus (CCV) in breeding kennels [12], and canine leptospirosis in outdoor hunting dogs [4].

Vaccines are differentiated into two categories based on whether the immunogen is live or inactivated (killed) [7]. Live vaccines have usually been attenuated by some process to render them avirulent when introduced into an immunocompetent animal. The process can include passage of the virus in cell cultures, temperature selection of mutants, and recombinant technology using vectors [4,7]. Killed vaccines have been inactivated by physical or chemical methods that destroy the infectivity but retain the immunogenicity necessary to induce a protective immune response. The advantages and disadvantages of live and inactivated vaccines are listed in Table 1.

VACCINE REGULATION

Extensive quality control measures have been established over the years to ensure that the vaccines used in human beings and animals are pure, safe, and efficacious [13–17]. Standards for animal vaccines are well outlined, and quality control is highly regulated by the US Department of Agriculture (USDA)–Animal and Plant Health Inspection Service (APHIS) [16]. Despite this scrutiny, there have been occurrences in which adventitious microorganisms, primarily viruses, have been known to enter vaccine production and become part of the vaccine on release (Fig. 1). The ways in which viruses enter into the vaccine production cycle have been reviewed extensively [7,18–23]. They include (1) contamination of the original viral seed stock used to prepare the vaccine, (2) contamination of the cell cultures used in production to amplify the known virus in the vaccine pool, and (3) contamination of the reagents used to propagate the cells being used to amplify the known virus for vaccine production. These are important points to consider and are discussed in further detail.

Contamination of the original viral seed stock would be when a known virus is being selected for eventual use in a vaccine. An example would be using an isolate of feline calicivirus that was derived from a cat with severe clinical symptoms. In the process of isolation, a passenger virus, such as feline panleukopenia, would also be isolated but not detected because of low virus titer or absence of cytopathologic findings. Usually, the virus being selected would be taken through steps to exclude passenger viruses by plaque purification

Table 1
Advantages and disadvantages of live (attenuated) virus and killed (inactivated) virus vaccines

	Advantages	Disadvantages
Live vaccines	Mode of action is most similar to natural infection	Possible reversion to virulence
	Multiply in host; induce range of immune responses	Possible contaminating viruses
	Duration of immunity is usually long lasting	Inference by other agents and passive antibody
	No adverse side effects to foreign protein	Storage problems (heating)
		Possible production of latency
		Possible induction of abortion
		Possible shedding to susceptible cohort
		Temporary immune suppression up to 2 weeks
Killed vaccines	Quite stable	Require large amounts of antigen or may not contain protective antigens
	Easy to produce	Reactions can develop to foreign proteins or adjuvants
		Immunity is usually short-lived; multiple boosters are required
		Do not produce local immunity
		May not inactivate all the agent
		Other agents that are resistant to inactivating agent may be present (eg, prions)
		May induce aberrant disease

Adapted from Tizard IR. The use of vaccines. In: Tizard IR, editor. Veterinary immunology: an introduction. 8th edition. Philadelphia: Saunders; 2008; with permission.

or limited dilution steps. Regulations required for vaccine production mandate seed stock purity, and vaccines must pass rigorous USDA standards referred to a 9 Code of Federal Regulations (9CFR) [16,17,23,24].

Examples of the latter two sources of contamination are more common and have been the most documented [21,22,24]. Contamination of cell cultures directly by latent noncytopathogenic viruses or indirectly by reagents used to propagate the cells in the laboratory involves several viruses (Table 2). Most common have been bovine viral diarrhea virus (BVDV), bovine and porcine parvoviruses, and bovine herpesvirus (BHV) type 4 [21,24]. These viruses are frequently present in fetal bovine serum, calf serum, bovine serum derivatives, and trypsin [21]. Although these viruses may have contaminated early serials of companion animal vaccines, there were no apparent serious clinical effects documented, because these viruses did not replicate in dogs or cats or, if replication did occur, there were no symptoms noted at safety testing. An exception to this may have been the association of BHV-4 with urinary tract disease in cats [25,26].

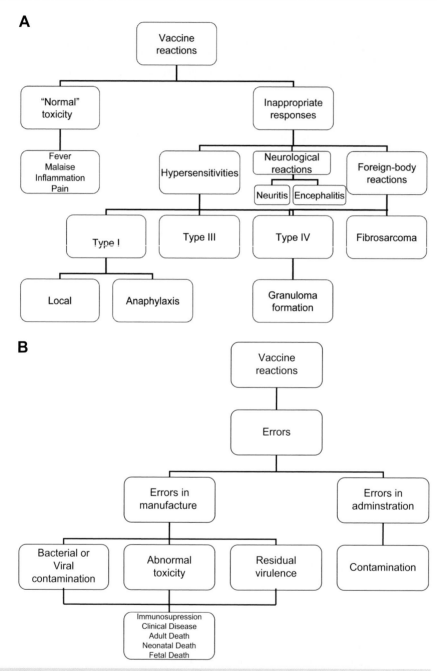

Fig. 1. The major adverse effects of vaccination. (A) Vaccine reactions result from normal toxicity and inappropriate responses from the host's immune system. (B) Vaccine reactions result from errors in manufacturing and administration. (Modified from Tizard IR. The use of vaccines. In: Tizard IR, editor. Veterinary immunology: an introduction. 8th edition. Philadelphia: Saunders; 2008. p. 276; with permission.)

Table 2
Specific viruses that are screened for in bovine serum (calf and fetal origin) and porcine trypsin used in production of veterinary biologics

Bovine serum	Trypsin
Adenovirus (groups 1 and 2)	Porcine adenoviruses
Akabane	African swine fever virus
Bovine coronavirus	Pseudorabies virus
Bovine ephemeral fever	Hemagglutinating encephalomyelitis virus
Bluetongue virus	Bovine viral diarrhea virus
Bovine leukosis	Hog cholera virus
Bovine immunodeficiency virus	Encephalomyocarditis virus
Bovine respiratory syncytial virus	Swine influenza virus
Bovine viral diarrhea virus	Porcine parvovirus
Rift valley fever virus	Porcine respiratory and reproductive syndrome
Vesicular stomatitis virus (Indiana and New Jersey)	Vesicular stomatitis virus (Indiana and New Jersey)
Bovine herpesviruses type 1, 2, 4	Transmissible gastroenteritis
Malignant catarrhal fever	Respiratory variant (coronavirus)
Parainfluenza virus type 3	Porcine enterovirus
Bovine polyomavirus	Vesicular exanthema virus
	Swine vesicular virus

Modified from Merten OW. Virus contamination of cell cultures—a biotechnological view. Cytotechnology 2002;39(2):101; with permission.

NOVEL CONTAMINATE WITH SERIOUS CONSEQUENCES

In 1992, a veterinarian noticed that pregnant dogs were aborting and, in some cases, the dam died as well. A common feature was a history of vaccination 3 to 4 weeks before whelping with a modified-live virus (MLV) multicomponent vaccine [27]. Initially, it was speculated that there was a component of the vaccine, such as canine parvovirus (CPV) type 2 or canine distemper virus (CDV), that was not properly attenuated and that because of the immune-compromised state of the dam, the virus was causing disease. Efforts to isolate CPV-2 and CDV were negative. A virus with properties of an orbivirus was isolated in cell culture from tissue homogenates derived from the diseased pups and dams, however [27,28]. The virus was eventually identified as bluetongue virus (BTV) type 11, a domestic strain of the virus common in the United States [28]. The veterinary biologic manufacturer and the National Veterinary Services Laboratory (NVSL) in Ames, Iowa were informed of the isolation of a potential viral contaminate. In subsequent testing by the NVSL, seed stock virus and repository samples were also found to be contaminated with BTV-11 [29]. The manufacturer voluntarily recalled all vials of the vaccine with serial numbers the same as those associated with the cases.

BTV had not previously been associated with disease in dogs but has been well documented as a pathogen of small and large ruminants [30]. The virus is now known to be present in serum products derived from these ruminants, such as fetal bovine serum. Subsequent studies have demonstrated that canine cells are capable of being infected with various serotypes of BTV, including BTV-11, without the cell cultures showing any cytopathologic change [31]. The aforementioned reports emphasized the importance of adding BTV detection methods to cells and virus seed stocks being used to produce companion animal vaccines.

ROLE OF VACCINES IN EMERGING VIRUSES

This is a controversial topic and has been debated in the literature over the past several decades [1,32–36]. There are several ways in which the vaccines may contribute to the emergence or re-emergence of viruses in the population. The first is by contaminated vaccines that are used routinely in a large percentage of the animal population. Vaccines that harbor adventitious agents for one species may be pathogenic for another species. Not only may the contaminated vaccine be pathogenic in the vaccinated animal, but it may be spread to other susceptible animals horizontally with the use of aerosols, feces, or saliva, for example (Fig. 2). Documentation of this form of cause and effect with a vaccine and emerging disease would need a thorough case history and laboratory data.

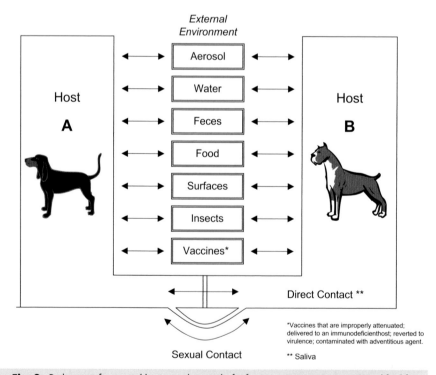

Fig. 2. Pathways of potential horizontal spread of infectious microorganisms. (*Modified from* DeFilippis VR, Villarreal LP. An introduction to the evolutionary ecology of viruses. In: Hurst CJ, editor. Viral ecology. San Diego (CA): Academic Press; 2000. p. 125–208; with permission.)

The second way in which vaccines may contribute to the emergence of new viruses is by immune selection of escape mutants (Fig. 3) [35,36]. Viruses are continually undergoing natural selection because they are obligate intracellular pathogens [37,38]. The immune response is evolving with the emergence of new viruses [39,40]. In some cases, it has been speculated that the use of vaccines causes an enhanced immune selection of viruses that evade the immune response, resulting in sustained infection in the population and disease in a certain percentage of the animals [35,36]. The immune response is a genetically adaptable system to microbial infections [39]. The appearance of new viral infections is most likely manifested first in immunocompromised animals, such as pregnant animals, neonates, and animals that are genetically immune deficient [41].

ENHANCED VIGILANCE: ROLE OF THE CLINICIAN
The emergence or re-emergence of a novel virus occurs in a clinical setting in which (1) well-vaccinated dogs or cats become diseased with clinical signs

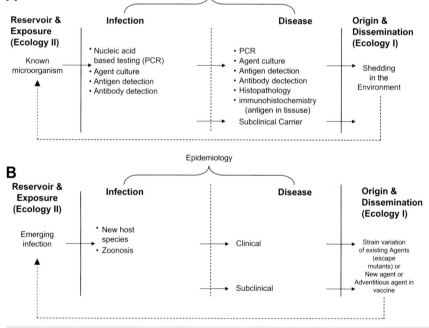

Fig. 3. Schematic of the relations between the epidemiology and ecology of an infectious microorganism. (A) Progression of infection to disease or subclinical carrier and the shedding into the environment. (B) Origin and dissemination of new microorganisms that emerge by means of mutation, recombination, or an adventitious microorganism in contaminated vaccine. (*Modified from* Evermann JF, Sellon RK, Sykes JE. Laboratory diagnosis of viral and rickettsial infections and epidemiology of infectious disease. In: Greene CE, editor. Infectious diseases of the dog and cat. 3rd edition. Philadelphia: WB Saunders; 2006. p. 8; with permission.)

resembling a virus that the animal should have been protected against by the vaccine, (2) a virus occurs in immunocompromised animals, or (3) a virus is rapidly introduced into a totally immunologically native population of dogs or cats [42]. The diseased animal should be quarantined, and a full diagnostic workup would proceed through a list of differentials [3,42–44]. If a well-vaccinated animal was clinically ill, a diagnostic pursuit would be made in parallel with contacting the biologic manufacturer, and the USDA, Center for Veterinary Biologics [45]. The two-page "Adverse Event Report" can be submitted on-line or faxed to 515-232-7120. This allows biologic manufacturers and the USDA to conduct postlicensure surveillance and to monitor the safety and efficiency of vaccines [9,13,16].

ENHANCED VIGILANCE: LABORATORY LEVEL
Testing for emerging or re-emerging viruses requires a familiarity with the common infectious agents affecting a particular species and maintaining an open mind for unusual observations, such as occurred in the BTV case mentioned previously [27]. The testing for novel viruses would have to be conducted on least at two levels. This would include testing that is done on biologics to ensure their purity before inoculation into animals [20,24] and testing that would be done at the diagnostic laboratory on diseased animals [33,46–49]. Virus-specific detection may involve (1) viral culture in susceptible noncontaminated cell lines, (2) viral antigen detection using immunofluorescence reagents, (3) viral antigen detection using ELISA; or (4) viral nucleic acid detection using polymerase chain reaction (PCR) [19,22,50,51].

DANGER OF CONTAMINATED VACCINES
The danger of a contaminated vaccine may include an immediate effect, such as the clinical effects that were reported after use of the multicomponent canine MLV that was contaminated with BTV [28]. The disease symptoms were confined to the inoculated dogs, and there was no evidence that further spread occurred to other potentially susceptible dogs in the vicinity. In this regard, the scenario would seem similar to the spread of some viruses to a dead-end or accidental host. This has been well documented for insect-borne viruses, such as West Nile virus, in isolated canine cases [48].

The long-term effects of a contaminated vaccine would be more difficult to document, and would require the availability of diagnostic assays specific for the adventitious virus. Because there is a certain degree of natural cross-species infection ("spill over") that occurs in the companion animal population, determining the origin of such an infection would require that the referring veterinarian work closely with the veterinary diagnostic laboratory with case history and sample submission (antemortem and postmortem) [42,52,53]. Once a virus were to spill over to another species, such as a cat to dog with feline calicivirus [46,54,55], the long-term danger is that the virus would establish the dog as a host, with subsequent virus replication, disease, and further shedding to susceptible dogs. This is postulated to have happened when feline panleukopenia virus crossed species in the late 1970s, resulting in CPV-2 [1,5]. This virus continues to circulate in the canine population, continues to have minor antigenic drifts (CPV-2a→CPV-2b→CPV-2c) [56], and has acquired a dual host range between dogs and cats [33,57].

SUMMARY

The use of biologics in veterinary medicine has been of tremendous value in safeguarding our animal populations from debilitating and oftentimes fatal disease. In parallel to the use of these biologics, there has been the continued evolution of new standards to maintain safety of the vaccines. This article reviewed the principles of vaccination and the extensive quality control efforts that are incorporated into preparing the vaccines. Examples of adverse events that have occurred in the past and how enhanced vigilance at the level of the veterinarian and the veterinary diagnostic laboratory help to curtail these events were discussed. Emphasis on understanding the ecology of viral infections in dogs and cats was introduced, together with the concepts of the potential role of vaccines in interspecies spread of viruses.

Acknowledgments

The author acknowledges the mentoring of Dr. Richard Ott and Dr. John Gorham. He thanks Dr. Linn Wilbur, Dr. Tom Baldwin, and Alison McKeirnan for their laboratory expertise. He expresses his appreciation to the practicing veterinarians who were instrumental in looking for adventitious microorganisms, particularly Dr. Vern Pedersen, Dr. Jeff Howlett, Dr. Charles Lohr, and Dr. Fineas Hughbanks. The author extends major thanks to Theresa Pfaff for assistance with manuscript preparation and Rich Scott for help with preparation of figures. His gratitude is extended to Linda Shippert for assistance with the literature review.

References

[1] Flint SJ. Evolution and emergence. In: Flint SJ, Enquist LW, Racanrello VR, et al, editors. Principles of virology: molecular biology, pathogenesis, and control of animal viruses. 2nd edition. New York: ASM Press; 2004. p. 759–802.

[2] Lutticken D, Segers RP, Visser N. Veterinary vaccines for public health and prevention of viral and bacterial zoonotic diseases. Rev Sci Tech 2007;26:165–77.

[3] Battersby I, Harvey A. Differential diagnosis and treatment of acute diarrhoea in the dog and cat. In Practice 2006;28:480–3.

[4] Greene CE, Schultz RD. Immunoprophylaxis. In: Greene CE, editor. Infectious diseases of the dog and cat. Philadelphia: Saunders; 2006. p. 1069–119.

[5] Prittie J. Canine parvoviral enteritis: a review of diagnosis, management, and prevention. J Vet Emerg Crit Care 2004;14:167–76.

[6] Speakman A. Management of infectious disease in the multi-cat environment. In Practice 2005;27:446–53.

[7] Tizard IR. The use of vaccines. In: Tizard IR, editor. Veterinary immunology: an introduction. 8th edition. Philadelphia: Saunders; 2008. p. 270–85.

[8] Thrusfield M. Companion animal health schemes. In: Thrusfield M, editor. Veterinary epidemiology. 3rd edition. Ames (IA): Blackwell Publ.; 2005. p. 379–81.

[9] Hustead DR, Carpenter T, Sawyer D, et al. Vaccination issues of concern to practitioners. J Am Vet Med Assoc 1999;214:1000–2.

[10] Moore GE, Glickman LT. A perspective on vaccine guidelines and titer tests for dogs. J Am Vet Med Assoc 2004;224:200–3.

[11] Thrusfield M. The control and eradication of disease vaccination. In: Thrusfield M, editor. Veterinary epidemiology. 3rd edition. Ames (IA): Blackwell Publ.; 2005. p. 386–7.

[12] Evermann JF, Abbott JR, Han S. Canine coronavirus—associated puppy mortality without evidence of concurrent canine parvovirus infection. J Vet Diagn Invest 2005;17:610–4.

[13] Dittmann S. Vaccine safety: risk communication—a global perspective. Vaccine 2001;19: 2446–56.

[14] Dory D, Gravier R, Jestin A. Risk assessment in new and conventional vaccines. Dev Biol (Basel) 2006;126:253–9.

[15] Grein K, Papadopoulos O, Tollis M. Safe use of vaccines and vaccine compliance with food safety requirements. Rev Sci Tech 2007;26:339–50.

[16] Meyer EK. Vaccine-associated adverse events. Vet Clin North Am Small Anim Pract 2001;31:493–514.

[17] Todd JI. Good manufacturing practice for immunological veterinary medicinal products. Rev Sci Tech 2007;l26:135–45.

[18] Day MJ. Vaccine side effects: fact and fiction. Vet Microbiol 2006;117:51–8.

[19] Duncan P, McKerral L, Feng S, et al. Detection breadth and limits for potential adventitious/ endogenous contaminants in biopharmaceutical processes: a reality check for innovative methods. Dev Biol (Basel) 2006;126:283–90.

[20] Evermann JF. Monitoring vaccines, diagnostic reagents and biotherapeutics for contaminating viruses. Br Vet J 1996;152:131–4.

[21] Merten OW. Virus contamination of cell cultures—a biotechnological view. Cytotechnology 2002;39(2):91–116.

[22] Ottiger HP. Monitoring veterinary vaccines for contaminating viruses. Dev Biol (Basel) 2006;126:309–19.

[23] Roth JA. Mechanistic basis for adverse vaccine reactions and vaccine failures. Adv Vet Med 1999;41:681–700.

[24] Black JW. Isolation of BVDV from bovine serum by EMEA/CVMP and 9 CFR: a comparison. Dev Biol (Basel) 2006;126:293–9.

[25] Goyal SM, Naeem K. Bovid herpesvirus-4: a review. Vet Bull 1992;62:181–201.

[26] Kruger JM, Osborne CA, Goyal SM, et al. Clinicopathologic and pathologic findings of herpesvirus-induced urinary tract infection in conventionally reared cats. Am J Vet Res 1990;51:1649–55.

[27] Evermann JF, McKeirnan AJ, Wilbur LA, et al. Canine fatalities associated with the use of a modified live vaccine administered during late stages of pregnancy. J Vet Diagn Invest 1994;6:353–7.

[28] Wilbur LA, Evermann JF, Levings RL, et al. Abortion and death in pregnant bitches associated with a canine vaccine contaminated with bluetongue virus. J Am Vet Med Assoc 1994;204:1762–5.

[29] Levings RL, Wilbur LA, Evermann JF, et al. Abortion and death in pregnant bitches associated with a canine vaccine contaminated with bluetongue virus. Dev Biol Stand 1996;88:219–20.

[30] Zientara S, Breard E, Sailleau C. Bluetongue: characterization of virus types by reverse transcription polymerase chain reaction. Dev Biol (Basel) 2006;126:187–96.

[31] Ianconescu M, Akita GY, Osburn BI. Comparative susceptibility of a canine cell line and bluetongue virus susceptible cell lines to a bluetongue virus isolate pathogenic for dogs. In Vitro Cell Dev Biol Anim 1996;32:249–54.

[32] DeFilippis VR, Villarreal LP. An introduction to the evolutionary ecology of viruses. In: Hurst CJ, editor. Viral ecology. San Diego (CA): Academic Press; 2000. p. 125–208.

[33] Ikeda Y, Nakamura K, Miyazawa T, et al. Feline host range of canine parvovirus: recent emergence of new antigenic types in cats. Emerg Infec Dis 2002;8:341–6.

[34] Nathanson N. Virus perpetuation in populations: biological variables that determine persistence or eradication. In: Peters CJ, Calisher CH, editors. Infectious diseases from nature: mechanisms of viral emergence and resistance. New York: Springer; 2005. p. 3–15.

[35] Radford AD, Dawson S, Wharmby C, et al. Comparison of serological and sequence-based methods for typing feline calicivirus isolates from vaccine failures. Vet Rec 2000;146: 117–23.

[36] Schat KA, Baranowski E. Animal vaccination and the evolution of viral pathogens. Rev Sci Tech 2007;26:327–38.

[37] Coyne KP, Reed FC, Porter CJ, et al. Recombination of feline calicivirus within an endemically infected cat colony. J Gen Virol 2006;87:921–6.

[38] Hurley KF, Pesavento PA, Pedersen NC, et al. An outbreak of virulent systemic feline calicivirus disease. J Am Vet Med Assoc 2004;224:241–9.

[39] Doherty PC, Turner SJ. The virus-immunity ecosystem. In: Peters CJ, Calisher CH, editors. Infectious diseases from nature: mechanisms of viral emergence and persistence. New York: Springer; 2005. p. 17–32.

[40] Marano N, Rupprecht C, Regenery R. Vaccines for emerging infections. Rev Sci Tech 2007;26:203–15.

[41] Evermann JF, McKeirnan AJ, Gorham JR. Interspecies spread of viruses between dogs and cats. Compendium of Continuing Education for the Practicing Veterinarian 2002;24: 390–6.

[42] Friend M. Disease emergence and resurgence. In: Friend M, Hurley JW, Nol P, et al, editors. Disease emergence and resurgence: the wildlife-human connection. Reston (VA): U.S. Dept of the Interior, U.S. Geological Survey; 2006. p. 19–126.

[43] Evermann JF, Sellon RK, Sykes JE. Laboratory diagnosis of viral and rickettsial infections and epidemiology of infectious disease. In: Greene CE, editor. Infectious diseases of the dog and cat. 3rd edition. Philadelphia: WB Saunders; 2006. p. 1–9.

[44] Evermann JF, Berry ES, Baszler T, et al. Diagnostic approaches for the detection of bovine viral diarrhea (BVD) virus and related pestiviruses. J Vet Diagn Invest 1993;5:265–9.

[45] APHIS, USDA. Available at: www.aphis.usda.gov/animal_health/vet_biologics. Accessed April, 2008.

[46] Evermann JF, McKeirnan AJ, Smith AW, et al. The isolation and identification of caliciviruses from dogs with enteric infections. Am J Vet Res 1985;46:218–20.

[47] Kramer JW, Evermann JF, Leathers CW, et al. Experimental infection of two dogs with a canine isolate of feline herpesvirus type I. Vet Pathol 1991;28:338–40.

[48] Lichtensteiger CA, Greene CE. West Nile virus infection. In: Greene CE, editor. Infectious diseases of the dog and cat. 3rd edition. Philadelphia: Saunders; 2006. p. 192–5.

[49] Mochizuki M, Hashimoto M, Roerink F, et al. Molecular and seroepidemiological evidence of canine calicivirus infections in Japan. J Clin Microbiol 2002;40:2629–31.

[50] Lau LT, Fung YW, Yu AC. Detection of animal viruses using nucleic acid sequence-based amplification (NASBA). Dev Biol (Basel) 2006;126:7–15.

[51] Vannier P, Espeseth D, editors. New diagnostic technology: applications in animal health and biologics control. Dev Biol 2006;126 [Switzerland: Karger].

[52] Vannier P, Capua I, LePotier MF, et al. Marker vaccines and the impact of their use on diagnosis and prophylactic measures. Rev Sci Tech 2007;26:351–72.

[53] Yoon KJ, Cooper VL, Schwartz KJ, et al. Influenza virus infection in racing greyhounds. Emerg Infect Dis 2005;11:1974–6.

[54] Evermann JF, Bryan GM, McKeirnan AJ. Isolation of a calicivirus from a case of canine glossitis. Canine Pract 1981;8:36–9.

[55] Evermann JF, McKeirnan AJ, Ott RL, et al. Diarrheal condition in dogs associated with virus antigenically related to feline herpesvirus. Cornell Vet 1982;72:285–91.

[56] Hong C, Decars N, Desario C, et al. Occurrence of canine parvovirus type 2c in the United States. J Vet Diagn Invest 2007;19:535–9.

[57] Truyen U, Evermann JF, Vieler E, et al. Evolution of canine parvovirus involved loss and gain of feline host range. Virology 1996;215:186–9.

ELSEVIER
SAUNDERS

Vet Clin Small Anim 38 (2008) 931–936

VETERINARY CLINICS
SMALL ANIMAL PRACTICE

INDEX

Note: Page numbers of article titles are in **boldface** type.

0195-5616/08/$ – see front matter
doi:10.1016/S0195-5616(08)00120-4